To Jack Babbitt Sr.

Thank you, Jack, for making our lives better.

# THE NEW THREAT OF TYPE 3 DIABETES

## Connecting High Blood Sugar Levels to Dementia and Alzheimer's Disease

Alan D. Raguso
Maria Lizotte, RN, BSN, CDE

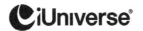

# THE NEW THREAT OF TYPE 3 DIABETES CONNECTING HIGH BLOOD SUGAR LEVELS TO DEMENTIA AND ALZHEIMER'S DISEASE

iUniverse books may be ordered through booksellers or by contacting:

iUniverse
1663 Liberty Drive
Bloomington, IN 47403
www.iuniverse.com
1-800-Authors (1-800-288-4677)

ISBN: 978-1-5320-5329-0 (sc)
ISBN: 978-1-5320-5328-3 (e)

Library of Congress Control Number: 2018909668

Print information available on the last page.

iUniverse rev. date: 10/31/2018

# Contents

Acknowledgments .................................................................................... ix

Introduction............................................................................................ xi

The Many Faces of Diabetes....................................................................1

The Body Chemistry Link to Major Diseases............................................3

The Links .................................................................................................5

Total Diabetes Warfare: The Means, the Will, and the Knowledge.......6

Just Coping with Diabetes Is Not Acceptable.......................................9

Maria's Personal Story of Type 1 Diabetes ...........................................10

pH Balance .............................................................................................11

Insulin Resistance ..................................................................................13

Prediabetes............................................................................................14

Type 1 Diabetes .....................................................................................15

Type 1.5 Diabetes ...................................................................................16

Type 2 Diabetes .....................................................................................18

Type 3 Diabetes .....................................................................................19

Tips to Avoid Glucose Spikes and Dawn Phenomenon ...................... 20

Glucose Bumps.......................................................................................21

Insulin Resistance and Glucose Variability ......................................... 22

The Food Groups ................................................................................... 24

The Three States of Carbohydrates...................................................... 28

A Matter of Balance............................................................................... 30

Diabetes Reversal Techniques...............................................................33

High-, Moderate-, and Low-Acid and Alkaline Foods and Beverages................35

The BEST Syndrome .............................................................................. 39

The Alkaline Diet ................................................................................... 43

The Mediterranean Anti-Inflammation Diet (MAID)........................... 45

Counting Processed Sugars and Carbohydrates.................................. 48

Pullout Quick Reference Guide ............................................................ 49

Minerals, Vitamins, and Micronutrients ...............................................51

Low-Carbohydrate Diets ....................................................................... 58

Glycemic Load.........................................................................................61

Maintaining Low Glucose Levels ..........................................................62

The Four Bs...........................................................................................64
The Three Ps..........................................................................................65
Stocking Your Food Arsenal ................................................................66
Low–Glycemic Load Foods ...................................................................69
Resistance Training and Weight Training to Reduce Insulin Resistance............70
Six Key Hormones You Should Know About .........................................72
Timing Is Everything ............................................................................74
Genetics and Biomarkers.......................................................................77
Convergence ..........................................................................................79
The Connection of Low pH Levels to Inflammation, Insulin
Resistance, and Type 2 and Type 3 Diabetes .........................................80
Processed Wheat, Gluten, Soy, and Sugars Can Be Toxic to Us ...........83
The Five Worst Foods to Eat .................................................................84
Senior Citizens and Type 3 Diabetes.....................................................85
The Keys to the Car ...............................................................................87
Questions and Answers..........................................................................88

Summary.................................................................................................91
Conclusion .............................................................................................93
Our Mission ...........................................................................................97
About the Author: Alan D. Raguso.........................................................99
About the Author: Maria Lizotte...........................................................101
Resources...............................................................................................103
Index .....................................................................................................107

# Illustrations

The Three Mirrors
The Chain
The Cover of *The Diabetes Slayer's Handbook*
The Steamroller
The Three Physical States of Carbohydrates
Reversing Diabetes Is a Matter of Balance
The Cucumber and the Pickle
High-, Moderate-, and Low-Acid and Alkaline Foods and Beverages
The Wall
The Bee
The "Safe" House
Pullout Quick Reference Guide
A1C to eAG Conversion Chart
The Turtle

# Acknowledgments

We would like to thank the following people:

Stace Filan for the book cover illustration; Allyson Filan for the interior illustrations; our doctors who never quit believing in us; Megan Eaton for the design work on the "Safe" House illustration; the diabetes educators of the Providence St. Mary Medical Center (PSMMC) Diabetes Education Department, Walla Walla, Washington; Son Bridge Community Center; and Alan's wife, Linda, for her interior illustrations and dedication to the production of this book.

Last but by no means least, we want to thank our fellow diabetes patients.

# Introduction

A few years ago, Alan D. Raguso published *The Diabetes Slayer's Handbook* as a motivational book to help fellow patients to understand and deal with prediabetes and type 2 diabetes. Over seven years ago, he made a commitment to change his life for the better. Later he became aware that he could help others by interacting with them in diabetes support group meetings and workshops. Eventually he started researching this disease called diabetes and became shocked as to what he perceived as a very misunderstood condition—misunderstood not only by patients but also by some medical professionals themselves. He has had the pleasure of being a member of the Providence St. Mary Medical Center advisory committee for diabetes education for the past five years and has participated in many support group meetings and workshops. It is an honor for him to be able to participate in helping others combat diabetes.

Several years ago he met Maria Lizotte, RN, BSN, CDE, when he made the first of many presentations of his Mediterranean anti-inflammation diet (MAID) and its illustrative form, the "Safe" House. Maria and Alan teamed together to hold education meetings for the On the Edge program at the local YMCA center for prediabetics. At these meetings they also accepted type 2 diabetics for the simple fact that these patients bring a lot to the table. The conventional thought was that mixing prediabetics together with type 2 diabetics would "confuse the patients." Contrary to that, Raguso and Lizotte found that once patients could understand the connections of this disease and how it affected so many, patients came away from meetings with a much better understanding of their medical condition and started asking their doctors and medical care providers questions—many questions.

On May 5, 2014, Alan and Maria founded the Diabetes Information Group (DIG). Their mission is simple. They want patients to be empowered to take charge of their condition of prediabetes or type 2 diabetes and come out winners. They accept type 1 and type 2 diabetics, as well as prediabetics and the families, friends, and caregivers for all these diabetics. All their meetings are free, as well as all the handouts. They do not ask for donations and don't need them. If there is a patient who can't afford to buy Alan's first book, Alan will give it to them free. Patients should not have to pay for critical medical knowledge!

Maria Lizotte is incredibly knowledgeable in the subject of diabetes. Being a type 1 diabetic herself for more than thirty years, she brings to the table personal experience along with her vast medical knowledge of the various forms of diabetes.

There is one thing that matters the most to both Alan and Maria: they truly care about their fellow patients improving their lives and enjoying life as it was meant to be, not being isolated and facing deteriorating health.

Alan and Maria give free lectures to various local organizations, and many of their attendees are elderly patients. Recently Maria started giving presentations at lectures of the condition known as type 3 diabetes. This is a new term being assigned to the conditions known as Alzheimer's disease and dementia. This new revelation connecting high blood sugar (glucose) levels to brain cognitive loss is riveting. Alan had been working on a second book relating to diabetes but changed direction midstream to deal with this topic. Maria agreed to coauthor with him on this new book. Her medical knowledge and background have been invaluable in creating this book.

Within ten years, the number of prediabetic and type 1 and type 2 diabetes patients, both diagnosed and undiagnosed in the United States, will be at about 30 percent, almost one-third, of the US population! Add to that an ever-increasing senior population, and the number of Alzheimer's disease and dementia patients, both diagnosed and undiagnosed, and the statistics are overwhelming.

Alan and Maria felt compelled to address the root cause of so many of these diseases the United States as a nation is combating. There are some root causes that lead to many of these diseases, and there are some ways to make simple changes in lives in order to live healthier, better, and longer.

This book will go through the various concepts of body chemistry and look at what really poses a tremendous health risk to everyone—*inflammation*. This condition is a result of exposure to wrong food intake, heredity, and environmental conditions, along with economics, poor pH (high acidity) balance, lack of moderate exercise, and our modern technological world. The book will carefully go through basic definitions of medical terms, the possible connection to prediabetes, type 2 and type 3 diabetes, and the steps you can take to prevent or reverse these diseases. All these diseases are connected to one another. In that sense, we are all in this war together!

Some illustrations and segments from *The Diabetes Slayer's Handbook: Preventing or Reversing Prediabetes and Type 2 Diabetes* will be used. Many concepts will be discussed. The authors like to use visual illustrations to help patients grasp concepts more quickly and more easily. One needs to understand and grasp the concepts of excess body sugar, acids as opposed to alkaline, and resulting inflammation, which can be as deadly as, or more deadly than, elevated levels of bad cholesterol (LDL). The book will discuss homocysteine levels in bad cholesterol readings. Hormones will be discussed in further detail than in the first book; Alan and Maria will discuss six key hormones. Exercise will be discussed in greater detail, and vitamins and supplements will be reviewed further.

Alan and Maria can't emphasize enough that patients need to talk with their doctors and health care providers, nutritional experts, dietitians, and physical trainers before implementing a new program or changing an existing program of nutrition or exercise. As much medical knowledge as Maria and Alan have, they still consult various medical experts for advice in their personal health journeys. Just remember that cutting-edge information is powerful but if used improperly can be dangerous and even catastrophic. Choose wisely and live wisely.

"The Three Mirrors" illustration is part of the pH balance concept, which involves phytonutrients that help combat heart disease, cancer, stroke, prediabetes, and type 2 and type 3 diabetes. Type 3 diabetes is the logical final step of the diabetes chain. It's time we understand all the implications we are facing.

# The Many Faces of Diabetes

Diabetes includes many different forms. Among these are the following:

- insulin resistance
- prediabetes
- type 1 diabetes
- type 1.5 diabetes
- type 2 gestational diabetes
- type 3 diabetes

## Type 1.5 Diabetes

Type 1.5 diabetes has two forms. It's often misdiagnosed as type 1 or type 2 diabetes.

The first form is LADA (latent autoimmune diabetes of adults).

The second form is MODY (maturity onset of diabetes in youth—though we now know adults get this also). One of the genetic types of MODY is seen in thin diabetics of any age. Currently only six genetic types can be tested for in the lab. Testing is very expensive but possible. Most insurance companies will not cover the cost. Persons at high risk of MODY include those who

- are of normal or thin weight but are diagnosed diabetic;
- are not helped by metformin, a low creative protein test;
- have fasting blood sugar over 125 that does not come down with diet, drugs, or insulin;
- have glucose in their urine with normal blood sugar levels; or
- have normal A1C after fasting but high postmeal blood sugars.

Testing markers include C peptide and antibodies.

### Type 2 Diabetes

Diabetes mellitus refers to type 2 diabetes, which used to be called adult onset diabetes until in recent years when more and more children and adolescents started developing the disease. So far nine different genes have been identified to cause this.

Patients are diagnosed with this if they have a fasting glucose over 100 and a maximum glucose reading of 140 two hours after a meal, with A1C readings in excess of 6.5.

### Gestational Diabetes

This is the type of diabetes that develops during pregnancy. Hormones released can increase insulin resistance in about 5 percent of women in this country. This condition usually develops in the third trimester and goes away after the baby is born. Be aware that about half of the women who have gestational diabetes develop type 2 diabetes later in life. Read *The Diabetes Slayer's Handbook* to learn how to prevent this.

### Type 3 Diabetes

This book will cover this newly termed form of diabetes resulting in some cases of dementia and Alzheimer's disease.

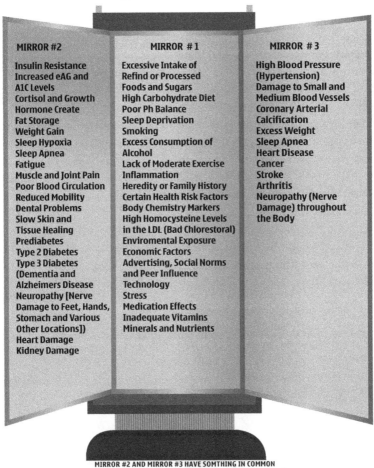

**MIRROR #2**

Insulin Resistance
Increased eAG and
A1C Levels
Cortisol and Growth
Hormone Create
Fat Storage
Weight Gain
Sleep Hypoxia
Sleep Apnea
Fatigue
Muscle and Joint Pain
Poor Blood Circulation
Reduced Mobility
Dental Problems
Slow Skin and
Tissue Healing
Prediabetes
Type 2 Diabetes
Type 3 Diabetes
(Dementia and
Alzheimers Disease
Neuropathy [Nerve
Damage to Feet, Hands,
Stomach and Various
Other Locations])
Heart Damage
Kidney Damage

**MIRROR #1**

Excessive Intake of
Refind or Processed
Foods and Sugars
High Carbohydrate Diet
Poor Ph Balance
Sleep Deprivation
Smoking
Excess Consumption of
Alcohol
Lack of Moderate Exercise
Inflammation
Heredity or Family History
Certain Health Risk Factors
Body Chemistry Markers
High Homocysteine Levels
in the LDL (Bad Chlorestoral)
Enviromental Exposure
Economic Factors
Advertising, Social Norms
and Peer Influence
Technology
Stress
Medication Effects
Inadequate Vitamins
Minerals and Nutrients

**MIRROR #3**

High Blood Pressure
(Hypertension)
Damage to Small and
Medium Blood Vessels
Coronary Arterial
Calcification
Excess Weight
Sleep Apnea
Heart Disease
Cancer
Stroke
Arthritis
Neuropathy (Nerve
Damage) throughout
the Body

MIRROR #2 AND MIRROR #3 HAVE SOMTHING IN COMMON
"THEY ARE REFLECTIONS OF THE CENTER MIRROR #1"
AUTHOR: ALAN D. RAGUSO COPYRIGHT 2015 ILLUSTRATED BY: ALAN D. RAGUSO

# The Body Chemistry Link to Major Diseases

Much like a chain, we can piece together the conditions and events that lead to major symptoms and diseases we wind up with as we grow older.

Please refer to the illustration labeled "The Three Mirrors." There are some things in mirror 1 that one can't have much control over, such as being born with a permanent lifetime condition or illness. Other factors, such as heredity or family history, along with certain body chemistry markers, environmental exposure (often unknown to the person affected), and general daily stress can be present and unchangeable. We might think we can control our daily stress, and to a degree we can, but for most of us, that is easier said than done. You may have often heard the phrase "life got in the way." How true it is that our best intentions often get trampled in the stampede of everyday survival and its stress.

Both of us, Alan and Maria, are here to tell you we understand. Just do your best. You can't ask for more. Doing your best varies each day.

Ask your doctor to check not just your LDL, or "bad" cholesterol, but the ratio of the "fluffy" LDL compared to the "dense" LDL, which is your real worry for heart disease.

Do all you can to talk with your doctor to determine that both you and he or she are doing everything within reason for you to stay healthy and avoid the conditions of prediabetes and type 2 and type 3 diabetes and their associated complications.

Remember—if you don't ask questions, you will never get answers.

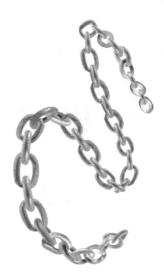

The Chain

Genetics, poor pH balance, high body acidity, IR (insulin resistance), prediabetes, type 2 diabetes, and type 3 diabetes.

# The Links

Please refer to "The Three Mirrors" illustration. You will see that conditions listed in the first mirror set up potential medical problems in the second mirror and serious medical conditions in the third mirror. Many of these final medical conditions can be life threatening.

Maintaining a healthy body chemistry can go a long way toward living a more pleasant and longer life.

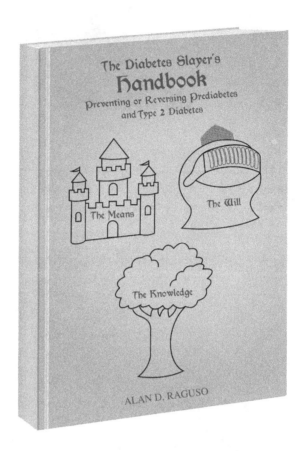

# Total Diabetes Warfare: The Means, the Will, and the Knowledge

There is no magical single pill, nutrient, vitamin, mineral, exercise technique, or dietary regime to defeat the various forms of diabetes. We see thousands of books professing "diabetes cures."

We need to clear the air about diabetes. It's heavily rooted in genetics, lifestyle, and environmental influences. Diabetes can be reversed, but it's never really gone. The propensity for diabetes is always still there. No one vitamin, food item, nutrient, or procedure will cure it. When we talk about reversing prediabetes or type 2 or type 3 diabetes, it must be remembered that diabetes can come back later with a vengeance.

When conducting warfare, the military employs all of its various assets to defeat an enemy. Implementing a limited strategy only gains limited success, not total victory. The enemy can come back to attack again later.

It's being revealed that there are many different types of diabetes, each with its own set of problems and ways needed to combat them.

When engaging the enemy diabetes, many different things have to be used in combination together to slow down the destructive effects of this disease. As mentioned in *The Diabetes Slayer's Handbook: Preventing or Reversing Prediabetes and Type 2 Diabetes*, this malady kills more than sixty thousand Americans per year. Both that book and this one are dedicated to friends of ours who were killed by this monster.

Diabetes is a terrorist. It will maim and kill as many people as possible just for fun. You do not negotiate with terrorists; total diabetes warfare is required. You take out a terrorist before it takes you out! As we have always said, "coping" with diabetes is not an acceptable option. Leaning back against an alley wall while a bully slowly beats you to a bloody pulp is not our idea of the way to cope with this disease. Our Steam Roller illustration demonstrates our resolve. You must be proactive, not reactive, when dealing with diabetes. You must go on the offensive and attack back. When the United States was attacked at Pearl Harbor in December 1941, we could have just "coped" with the situation and *negotiated* for peace. We did not negotiate. We went on one of the largest military offensives in history to preserve our health, welfare, and way of life. Do you want to give up your way of life? Of course not!

The cover of our first book, *The Diabetes Slayer's Handbook: Preventing or Reversing Prediabetes and Type 2 Diabetes*, has three images: a castle, a helmet, and a tree. A local newspaper article describing the book said those items were weapons. Actually they are not.

They are defensive in nature.

A strong castle not only is a place to be secure in, but it extends a message to your enemy: "Don't mess with me!"

A helmet, once again, is defensive in nature.

Finally, the last image is the tree of knowledge. Knowledge is powerful. In itself it does not act as an offensive weapon. There are those who fear the idea of others being given knowledge because it can free those others from the control of those who want power and control over them.

Each diabetic person must identify their illness, whether it be insulin resistance, prediabetes, or type 1, type 2, or type 3 diabetes. Then each person must seek out the advice of medical experts, counselors, and educators to learn how to immediately go on the defensive and then take the offensive to the disease.

Often we tend to ask the question, "Why me?" Our answer would be, "Why not?" What is important is not why something has affected us but how we deal with it.

When you feel alone battling a potentially life-threatening disease, it's easy to want to give up. Seek companionship with family, friends, and others who have similar medical conditions. Remember that when you help others, you help yourself. There is always someone out there who is in worse shape than you.

Total diabetes warfare is a concept suggesting that patients must take control of their destinies in life. Ultimately we determine our journeys through life. We realize there are things in life we can't control; however, there are a lot of things we can control.

Sometimes we need to hear things we don't want to hear. We need to do some self-analysis of ourselves; our mental outlook, philosophy, and faith can often guide us if we let them. Remember—when you have a little voice speaking in your head guiding you, *listen to the voice.*

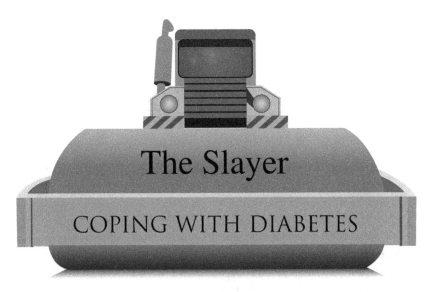

**The Steamroller**

# Just Coping with Diabetes Is Not Acceptable

We fully realize that dealing with diabetes can at times be depressing. We would suggest that you periodically visit a hospital or nursing home; there you will probably find patients far worse off than you are. Don't get isolated and start feeling alone and sad. Our illustration above shows a pavement roller, and the image is not meant to make light of the condition of diabetes; it is meant to send a message—fight! Some days we have setbacks, but that does not mean we give up. We the authors have had setbacks, but we keep going. There is a larger, bigger-than-life purpose for us to fulfill.

Once again, let us stress that if you help others and participate in diabetes group activities, you will feel better and have a much better outlook on life. Let's face it—we are all going to die. The big question is when. It's up to us to fill in the spaces in our journey through life. Think good thoughts.

# Maria's Personal Story of Type 1 Diabetes

Maria Lizotte has a bachelor's degree in nursing from the University of Pittsburgh and has been a nurse educator since 1993.

As a youngster with type 1 diabetes, her experience at diabetes camps inspired her to become a certified diabetes educator. She learned firsthand the power of diabetes education in improving day-to-day life.

Juvenile diabetes is a life-threatening, chronic disease.

Insulin is not a cure; it is just a Band-Aid.

Vigilance 24-7 is needed to avoid death from insulin shock or diabetic coma.

A funny thing: when she was diagnosed in the 1980s, she was not allowed to exercise alone, and intense exercise was not advised!

Having lived most of her life with the disease, Maria has a unique understanding of what people with diabetes live with, as well as a desire to share her knowledge to aid others living with the disease.

Whether you have prediabetes or have already been diagnosed with diabetes, Maria believes knowledge is the power to improve your quality of life with this disease.

# pH Balance

The term *pH* comes from the German word *poltzen*, meaning "power," and the periodic table symbol for the element hydrogen (H). The element hydrogen is the most common one in the universe. It makes up a massive amount of all the things around us, and indeed, we ourselves consist of vast quantities of this element. Hydrogen contains ions, which are positively or negatively charged. The positively charged hydrogen ions are the villains, and the negatively charged ions are the good guys.

Have you ever been in a swimming pool where the chemicals "weren't balanced" and the feel and smell of the water was not pleasant? Were you ever in a swimming pool that was crystal clean, fresh-smelling, and silky to the touch? In a sense, our bodies have to be kept balanced, much like a swimming pool, in order to operate properly. Basic chemistry consists of three states. They are the acid, alkaline, and neutral states. When you read a pH scale, 7.5 is the neutral state. Tap water is around 7.5 on the pH scale. The lower the number, the more acidic the condition of an object. Sulfuric acid would be at the bottom of the scale. The higher the number, the more alkaline (antacid) the condition. Soda ash would be high on the pH scale. Generally the pH scale will go to 15.0.

Once you can understand and maintain a good pH balance in your body, your health will start to improve dramatically.

Certain proteins accelerate fat loss.

Overacidity triggers weight gain.

Body tissue is "corroded," resulting in internal inflammation that damages vital organs such as the heart. The body's first line of defense is to pack on fat to fight rising acid levels.

Lemons contain organic acids, which give them a tart taste, but when this citrus fruit is consumed, it forms alkaline compounds that work to neutralize toxic acids in the body. Have a dietary intake of 80 percent alkaline-forming foods and limit intake of acid-forming foods (meat, dairy products, and bad carbohydrates) to 20 percent.

Natural sugar has no effect on hydrogen ions, yet once sugars start to be refined or processed, they become acidic and will cause damage to our bodies if consumed in large quantities. The key to good pH balance is countering acids with alkalines. For example, if you have eaten a pickle, then eat a cucumber. Oddly this is the same food, one natural and one processed. Refined and processed foods will be more acidic. Processed sugars and processed sugar substitutes are highly acidic yet natural. Stevia is highly alkaline.

The concept of pH balance goes hand in hand with the Mediterranean anti-inflammation diet (MAID). Many foods change pH composition when they are consumed. For example, lemon and lime juices are acidic, yet when consumed, they become alkaline in our bodies and not only slow the absorption of sugars into our bloodstream but also help increase the pH level in our bodies, which is a good thing!

Later we include tables of foods in six categories: high-, moderate-, and low-acid content foods and beverages, along with high-, moderate-, and low-alkaline foods and beverages.

Our journey through this book will show you the long chain of events that can lead to excess acidity in our bodies. Combined with inflammation and insulin resistance, such acidity will eventually result in serious health problems.

The control of low-pH foods and beverages, which include refined sugars, is key to preventing insulin resistance, prediabetes, and type 2 and type 3 diabetes. Cancer cells cannot survive or replicate in a high-pH environment. Vessels won't be prone to becoming inflamed and damaged in a good pH environment.

The more natural the foods you eat are, the higher the pH factor they will have. Once again we are back to the basics. "Eat what your grandparents ate!"

# Insulin Resistance

Insulin resistance is the precursor to prediabetes. Many things, including but not limited to inflammation, can cause this condition. The three-mirrors illustration in this book shows the progression from inflammation to insulin resistance and then to type 2, type 1.5, and type 3 diabetes. A person could develop type 3 diabetes without having previously developed the other types of diabetes.

Prediabetes, type 2 diabetes, excess weight, high blood pressure, high LDL (bad cholesterol), low HDL (good cholesterol), and high triglycerides levels combine to create "metabolic syndrome." Basically you're getting painted into a corner with multiple risks.

We have found that the majority of prediabetes and type 2 diabetes patients who are referred to diabetes counseling, diabetes workshops, diabetes support group meetings, and prediabetes combined exercise and education programs have been newly diagnosed with their condition, have control problems, or have risk factors that refer to metabolic syndrome.

# Prediabetes

The category of prediabetes should be considered a huge warning flag. In people with prediabetes, fasting glucose levels are above 100 mg/dl but lower than 126 mg/dl. Nonfasting glucose levels are above 140 mg/dl but lower than 200 mg/dl. The A1C is above 5.7 percent but lower than 6.5 percent.

Even at just prediabetic levels, people run the risk of serious complications of nerve disease, eye disease, circulation problems, kidney disease, and even heart attack, stroke, or amputation of toes, feet, and legs.

Health guidelines regarding prediabetes over the past years have treated the condition as a concern but not a serious threat. That is not the case! Together with your health care professionals, you can work to reverse your prediabetes condition.

If you have not had your glucose levels checked, you need to do so immediately! Prediabetes and the various forms of type 2 diabetes, including type 1.5 diabetes and type 3 diabetes, as well as dementia and Alzheimer's disease, are on the rise.

Steps need to be taken to protect your future health, quality of life, and longevity.

# Type 1 Diabetes

Type 1 diabetes is an autoimmune disease in which the body attacks and kills off the beta cells of the pancreas that make insulin. Only 5 percent of those with diabetes have this autoimmune type of the disease, and for such patients, insulin injection is needed for life. While most of the new diagnoses of this type of diabetes are seen in children under the age of five, it can develop even in older adults. Onset of this disease is fast, and it can be fatal if missed. In early 2015 two small children in different states were misdiagnosed with the flu. A simple urine test would have saved their lives.

# Type 1.5 Diabetes

Type 1.5 diabetes has two forms. It's often misdiagnosed as type 1 or type 2 diabetes.

The first form is LADA: latent autoimmune diabetes of adults.

Another autoimmune type of diabetes, the autoimmune part of this disease develops slowly, and it can take three to five years for a person to lose function of the beta cells that produce insulin. With this disease seen in adults over age thirty-five, it is not uncommon to be misdiagnosed, as it shares characteristics of both type 1 and type 2 diabetes. Diagnosis is vital: if type 2 medications are given that stimulate the beta cells to produce insulin, the autoimmune attack is fast-forwarded. Eating a low-carbohydrate diet will help delay the onset of complete beta cell failure. Some signs this might be your diagnosis are having another autoimmune disease, normal or near normal weight, or a family member with type 1 diabetes.

The second form is MODY: maturity onset of diabetes in the young.

This is a genetic cause of diabetes often seen in those with normal weight. We now know it can occur at any age, not just the young, and it is caused by one of nine possible genes. Many people diagnosed with type 2 diabetes may actually have the MODY gene. Scientists are currently discovering more genetic variables of MODY, and it is an evolving subject.

Type 1.5 diabetes can also be caused by other unknown genetic causes or environmental toxins.

Persons with normal weight and good insulin sensitivity but higher blood sugars and diagnosed as having type 2 diabetes are currently under research showing there are other genetic variables that cause this form of diabetes. There is also a theory that environmental toxins cause type 2 diabetes. These toxins are described as endocrine disruptors and are still being studied, but we do know that chemicals from plastics are one risk for type 2 diabetes, so avoid plastic water bottles.

No matter what your type of diabetes, high blood sugars are the end cause of all damage to the body and brain. No matter how high your blood sugars are running right now, you can get the level down and stop the damage from this point on.

# Type 2 Diabetes

Diabetes mellitus refers to type 2 diabetes, which used to be called adult onset diabetes until in recent years more and more children and adolescents started developing the disease.

Patients are diagnosed with this if they have a fasting glucose under 120 and a maximum glucose reading of 140 two hours after a meal. In addition, conventional A1C readings should be under 7.0. More aggressive guidelines call for a fasting glucose under 100 and a maximum glucose reading of 120 two hours after a meal. These guidelines specify that A1C readings should be under 6.5.

The vast majority of diabetics in the type 2 diabetes category can improve their health through diet and exercise. However, not all patients with type 2 diabetes are overweight. Excess weight may be a contributing factor to this condition, but there are many other factors that can affect it. Some patients are over two times their normal body weight but do not have type 2 diabetes! There are many other factors that influence type 2 diabetes, such as genetics, family history, environmental influences, stress, lack of exercise, poor eating habits, and even medications.

# Type 3 Diabetes

This condition refers to some cases of dementia and Alzheimer's disease, where excess levels of blood sugar (glucose) have caused long-term cognitive memory loss. Not all cases of dementia and Alzheimer's disease can be linked exclusively to high blood sugar levels.

Many cases of type 2 and type 3 diabetes can be traced back to the following conditions: excessive processed carbohydrates and sugars, high-carbohydrate diet, insulin resistance, poor pH balance, smoking, excess consumption of alcohol, lack of moderate exercise, inflammation, genetics (heredity), family history of risk factors, genetic markers, biomarkers, high homocysteine levels of bad cholesterol (LDL), environmental exposures, economic factors, social influences and norms, advertising, peer influence, and technology.

# Tips to Avoid Glucose Spikes and Dawn Phenomenon

It is very important to regulate your postmeal glucose levels after dinner at night. High glucose levels at night can continue until you get up the next morning. That's a lot of hours of high glucose levels. There goes your A1C level!

Read your food labels. You can't control the amount of sugar hitting your bloodstream if you don't have any idea how many grams of refined carbohydrates and sugars you're consuming. If you load up heavy on foods that convert to blood sugar quickly, of course you will get a glucose spike.

One of the biggest mistakes we all can make is simply consuming too much food in the evening and in particular too much of the wrong food later in the evening. We're setting ourselves up for a real ugly glucose reading in the morning.

You can get your muscle and tissue cells to be less insulin resistant using chlorophyll and burn more sugar with increased metabolism. And if you time and control the consumption of processed carbohydrates and sugars, you will see surprising and fast changes occur in your glucose readings. This sounds like trickery on your body. So what if it is? All's fair in war. Remember—you are at war with diabetes, and you want to come out the winner, not the loser.

# Glucose Bumps

A glucose bump is an increase of blood glucose by twenty-one to forty-nine points. A glucose spike is an increase of fifty or more points of blood glucose. Glucose bumps can pack on weight as badly as insulin spikes.

Here are three ways to ward off glucose bumps:

- Avoid high-fructose corn syrups, which cause a 48 percent weight gain and also elevate glucose.
- Avoid excess caffeine; drinking four to five cups a day elevates glucose.
- Magnesium can reduce insulin levels by 21 percent in four weeks. The pancreas does not need to pump out excess insulin. Be aware that magnesium can reduce your calcium levels, so talk to your doctor about taking a calcium supplement along with your magnesium supplement.

# Insulin Resistance and Glucose Variability

What is insulin resistance? Think of the hormone insulin, which the body produces for a specific function. The job of insulin is to go out into the body and ask the cells to open up to accept blood sugar. The insulin makes the call to the cells, and most of the time, they open the doors and let the blood sugar in. Sometimes the cells get inflamed or irritated by chemicals or toxins in the blood system, and they start having trouble picking up the phone call from the insulin. After a while this may result in metabolic syndrome and insulin resistance. The two terms are often used interchangeably; that is, metabolic syndrome is often referred to as insulin resistance.

An alkaline diet helps reverse insulin resistance. *Glucose variability* is a term used for a course of glucose going up and down each day for patients. The A1C test gives a general average of a person's glucose levels over a period of time and is generally a pretty good indicator of glucose tolerance. If you are prediabetic or have type 2 diabetes, this blood test will be conducted every three to six months depending on a patient's history of glucose tolerance. This test does not account for variations in the blood sugar level caused by gluten bumps (glucose elevated by twenty-one to forty-nine points) or glucose spikes (glucose elevated by fifty or more points). This concept of glucose variability can be more important than the A1C test itself.

Glucose variability may be as important as, if not more important than, the A1C measurement.

Glucose variability is the opposite of glucose stability. Instead of averaging the glucose levels over a period of at least ninety days, it takes into account the highs and lows of the glucose throughout the day. You want to avoid a roller coaster effect, with your blood sugar levels constantly going high and low and not being stabilized.

How can one check the variations or fluctuations in their glucose? The answer is to test, test, and test your glucose daily. For many this is difficult since they may not be covered for any more than fifty test strips *per month*. The first thing to do is have your doctor go to bat for you to get you authorized with your insurance company to get the number of test strips you need to be covered. You could get as many as five strips per day covered by your insurance company. If you are on a Medicare Advantage insurance plan, you might be able to get it done through them. Your doctor can argue a case that you are concerned your glucose is not staying stable enough and you need more strips to properly monitor your glucose readings.

Let's be blunt. We are all paying high medical insurance premiums and have paid heavily over the years into our Medicare and Social Security funds. You have the *right* to ask for or even demand service and adequate prescription coverage to maintain good health.

Insulin resistance is the precursor of prediabetes. It's our first warning flag that something is wrong. Heed the warning!

Prescription drugs can cause insulin resistance; statins are one possible source of elevated glucose resistance.

A high-alkaline diet helps *reverse* insulin resistance.

# The Food Groups

There are many ways to categorize food into groups. The most important breakdown for those with diabetes is the following.

## Carbohydrates

Carbohydrates consist of sugar (unrefined and refined) fiber, other fibers, and sugar alcohols.

You will often hear of the "starchy" foods. These foods are quick to break down into sugars after being eaten if they are heavily cooked and/or processed. Included in this category are breads, cereals, and grains, as well as potatoes, crackers, chips, snack foods, and legumes (the pod family), such as beans, peas, and lentils. I am not afraid to consume legumes when they are in their natural "dense" carbohydrate form. They will turn to sugar much more slowly. Avoid packaged products with added flavoring, cheeses, and sauces. That's where you can get into trouble with glucose control.

Carbohydrates basically break down into sugars, fiber, sugar alcohols, and other carbohydrates. I group carbohydrates into two groups: spikers (a spike is a glucose-reading increase greater than fifty), which rapidly turn into blood sugar, and stabilizers, which are slow to be absorbed into the bloodstream.

## Fruits

Fruits in their natural raw form, quick-frozen fruits, and canned fruits without sugar will do well for your health and reversing your diabetes. I eat virtually no canned fruits, even if they are in natural fruit juices instead of light, medium, or heavy added syrups. They still turn to sugar quicker because they have been precooked and thus some of the digestive process has already been eliminated.

Avoid fruit juice, which is high in sugar and low in fiber. Drink "diet" fruit juices, which are high in flavor and ultralow in carbohydrates and calories. There are extremely low-carbohydrate and low-calorie fruit beverages out there to enjoy, and they won't spike your glucose.

## Milk

While milk has a lot of nutrients, it is high in carbohydrates and calories. Compare the food labels of milk and unsweetened almond beverages. You will be shocked.

## Sweets, Desserts, and Other Carbohydrates

Travel through this one like you were walking through a minefield—*very carefully!*

## Nonstarchy Vegetables

These are at the top of the list for the MAID program. Green leafy vegetables are almost devoid of any carbohydrates and are loaded with chlorophyll. They also have substantial amounts of fiber in them that help you slow the absorption of sugar and give you a feeling of fullness. And yes, even the lowly iceberg lettuce plays a part in the battle plan to defeat diabetes.

## Proteins

Meat, fish, and nuts give you the building blocks to repair tissue. Also, they slow the absorption of sugar into your bloodstream.

## Fats

We eat plenty of good fats—in particular, omega-3 fats. We avoid the bad omega-6 fats.

## Alcohol

We limit the intake of alcohol drastically.

Experts recommend that you consume about 120 to 160 grams of carbohydrates per day. We're fine with that. What we do is limit our daily amount of processed carbohydrates to 30 grams per day. The rest of our carbohydrates are natural, dense carbohydrates that are slow to break down into sugar. When we read a food label, our first three concerns are

- the amount of net digestible carbohydrates,
- the amount of calorie content in the food serving, and
- the saturated (bad) fat content.

These are important for people when they read food labels.

Once again I want we emphasize that the MAID is not a low-carbohydrate diet. It's the type and quantity of certain types of carbohydrates that we consume that make the difference. Also, we eat plenty of healthy fats and protein. This system also is not low fat and not high protein. You need to keep your body balanced day after day.

This is not a sprint to achieve miraculous results in ninety days. Yes, you will see some results immediately, but remember this is a marathon for the rest of your life. This is a lifestyle *transition*. You gradually make changes that you can stay with and live with the rest of your life.

# THE THREE PHYSICAL STATES OF CARBOHYDRATES

## WATER IN 3 STATES

 VAPOR

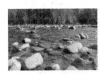 LIQUID

 ICE

## CARBOHYDRATES IN 3 STATES

 APPLE JUICE

 APPLESAUCE

 (RAW) UNPEELED APPLE

**Refined or (Processed) Carbs**
**HIGH GLYCEMIC LOAD**

Refined granulated sugars, Cane &
Sugar Beet (refined),
Processed White Rice,
Refined Breads

**Starches Moderate Carbs**
**MODERATE GLYCEMIC LOAD**

Squash-Butternut, Acorn Winter
100% Whole Wheat Bread, Long Grain White Rice.
Processed Grains, Corn, Potatoes,
Hominy, Peas

**Natural Dense Carbs**
**LOW GLYCEMIC LOAD**

Cooked whole grains, Oats,
(steel cut & rolled). Barley,
Brown Rice, Green Leafy Vegetables,
Zuchinni(squash), Brocolli, Jicama,
Spinach, Kale, Mushrooms, Onions,
Fresh Fruit, Blueberries, Apples,
Watermelon, Strawberries, Nuts,
Whole uncooked Grains.

There are"fast" carbohydrates which break
down rapidly into sugar in the bloodstream.
There are"moderate" carbohydrates that break¬
down slower and can be further slowed from
releasing sugar into the bloodstream by fiber,
good fats, acidic foods and low resistance interval
training and moderate resistance training exercise.
The dense natural carbs are <u>extremely slow</u> to be
converted into sugar in the bloodstream and if handled
"the right way" virtually won't be absorbed as sugar at all!

**\*\*GLUCOSE "BUMPS" 21 - 49
POINTS CAUSED BY STARCH
AND MODERATE
CARBOHYDRATES\*\***

**NOTE:** Lime, Lemon and Grapefruit juices **Neutralize sugar** and most Amazingly
they **Reduce** the acidity in our bodies, helping raise our PH levels to a healthy 7.0 + %!

www.thediabetesslayershandbook.com     Author ALAN D RAGUSO     Copyright 2012

# The Three States of Carbohydrates

Many people find understanding carbohydrates very complicated. We have worked to simplify the concept of carbohydrates for patients. Once you gain a good foothold of knowledge in that area, you will be able to navigate in the world of foods and beverages much more easily and with greater success.

Please refer to our illustration on the previous page showing the three physical states of carbohydrates. It splits carbohydrates into three basic categories. The illustration uses the concept of the three states of water as a comparison; water exists in three states: vapor, liquid, and solid. The vapor is light and moves easily; the liquid has some solid form but still can move. Ice is very solid, and it takes effort to break it apart. Such are carbohydrates; low-density "fast" carbohydrates are absorbed quickly in the form of sugar into our body. If you were experiencing hypoglycemia or extremely low blood sugar, drinking apple juice would elevate your glucose level quickly. Applesauce would be a somewhat denser carbohydrate, converting to sugar relatively quickly but not as rapidly as the apple juice. Lastly, the whole natural apple, when consumed, would convert to sugar much more slowly since it is a dense, natural carbohydrate. It is compared to solid ice as a form of water.

You will at times read about fast, moderate, and slow carbohydrates, which is a similar view of this categorization.

Many foods are in the form of starches, which is a moderate or semidense carbohydrate form. Starches can contain a lot of latent stored sugars, which eventually will convert into blood sugar (glucose) somewhat slower than faster converting carbohydrates, but nonetheless will turn into blood sugar. Many squashes, flours, potatoes, grains (e.g., rice, wheat, barley, and oats), and sweet potatoes have that ability to eventually convert into blood sugar. The more refined or processed the product is, the faster it will convert to sugar. Remember many processed or refined (manufactured) foods also have added sugar, salt, and preservatives, which can further expand the effect of sugar in the bloodstream. If your body cannot get the sugar taken in by the body's cells or expelled out, it will linger in your body, highly acidic, and eventually cause damage to your blood vessels and soft tissues. Diabetes loves soft targets.

## Where Are Carbohydrates Found?

Starches include the following:

> flour (cereal, bread/grains, pasta, crackers, tortillas)
> rice (cereal, rice, rice cakes)
> beans (all except green beans)
> corn (cereal, popcorn, tortillas)
> potatoes
> peas

one cup of milk = fifteen grams of carbohydrates

## What Is a Serving Size?

| |
|---|
| **Starch** 1/2 cup 15 grams carbohydrate<br>palm size 15 grams carbohydrate<br><br>**Pasta/Rice** 1/3 cup 15 grams carbohydrate |
| **Fruit** 1 cup 15 grams carbohydrate<br>fist size 15 grams carbohydrate<br>1/2 cup canned 15 grams carbohydrate |
| **Vegetable** 3 cups raw 15 grams carbohydrate<br>1 1/2 cup cooked 15 grams carbohydrate |

To see what works for you, check your blood glucose two hours after the meal.

Maria Lizotte RN, BSN, CDE 2002

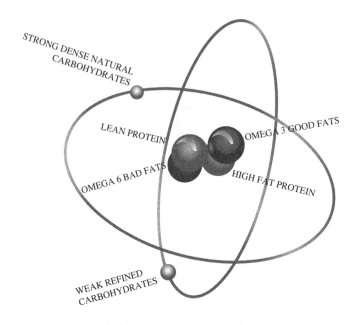

# A Matter of Balance

Throughout our book we consistently talk about balance. In essence we spend our entire lives maintaining a balancing act between our personal needs, our job, and social and family commitments we've made. The last thing that we usually are concerned about is balancing our personal life. Yet sometimes we have to put ourselves first when it comes to maintaining good health, which includes physical, emotional, and mental health. If we are nervous wrecks eating poorly, dashing about texting and talking on our cell phones, emailing, driving everywhere, and sleeping irregular hours, we shouldn't be surprised that our health begins to fade.

The previous page has a diagram of a helium atom isotope. This illustration shows the importance of combining low-resistance interval training, weight training, balance training, and resistance exercise with the other elements found circling and connected together. Without protons, electrons, and neutrons properly balanced, the atom would fall apart. The same case can be made for balancing lean protein with high-fat protein, good omega-3 fats and bad omega-6 fats, and of course dense natural carbohydrates and poor refined or processed carbohydrates.

When you look at the concept of having a balanced pH level in your body, this once again goes hand in hand with the Mediterranean anti-inflammation diet idea of balance and the alkaline diet concept of balance.

We do not recommend that any patient go off the deep end with a dietary program they can't maintain all their life. Yes, you need to commit to a healthy lifestyle for the rest of your life. You must find a way to improve your life, but in a way that you can sustain for the rest of your life.

Let's think of our term *total diabetes warfare*. Past the concept of a full-out assault, there's another concept to remember: intelligence, recon, and information gathering to help you eventually defeat your enemy.

In the case of diabetes, one has to spend time thinking about how we will overcome diabetes. When we talk about insulin resistance, prediabetes, type 1 and type 2 diabetes, and dementia and Alzheimer's disease (type 3 diabetes), if a shiver goes up your back, it should. These conditions lead to reduced quality of life, debilitation, exorbitant medical costs, strains on family and friends, and ultimately death caused by diabetes-related damage to the heart, kidneys, eyes, arteries, and yes, even the brain as we are now finding out.

We, the authors, have together fought both type 1 and type 2 diabetes for years. Both of us have done years of extensive research and have found that conventional medical theories run behind the science discoveries by about ten years.

If you embark on health changes in your life, consult your doctors, pharmacist, dietitian, medical caregivers, personal physical trainers, and therapists.

At all costs, get balance into your life!

The Cucumber and the Pickle
Both are the same food item
One is Alkaline
One is Acidic

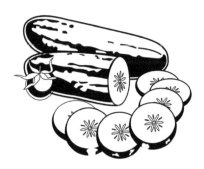

**ALKALINE**

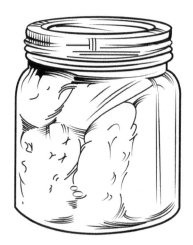

**ACIDIC**
The Cucumber and the Pickle

# Diabetes Reversal Techniques

As you have probably noticed, our food list contains items that are both low in processed carbohydrates and sugars and are gluten-free. If patients use the system correctly, it's almost impossible to fail. Between slowing and blocking the carbohydrates from being absorbed plus burning and neutralizing sugars and cranking the metabolism to 24-7, it's a deadly one-two punch to both obesity and diabetes. An increased intake of chlorophyll (eating green) helps to greatly reduce insulin resistance by getting the cells to operate to reduce cell inflammation and swelling. Add low-resistance interval training, and you should start feeling better immediately.

### Repair the faulty blood sugar control system.

This is done simply by substituting the pristine-looking but toxic mix of fats and oils found in plastic containers on your supermarket shelves with clean, healthy, beneficial fats and oils. Consume only flax oil, coconut oil, fish oil, and occasionally cod liver oil until blood sugars begin to stabilize. Then add back healthy oil, such as olive oil. Read labels; refuse to consume cheap junk oils when they appear in processed foods or on restaurant menus. Diabetics are chronically short of minerals. They need to add a good-quality, broad-spectrum mineral supplement to the diet.

### Control blood sugar manually during the recovery cycle.

Develop natural blood sugar control by the use of glycemic tables, by consuming frequent small meals (known as grazing) that include fiber-rich foods, and by regular after-meal exercise such as a walk, biking, resistance training, or some sort of light exercise you like. You want to avoid processed sugars, using only nontoxic sweeteners like stevia.

Restore a healthy balance of healthy fats and oils when the blood sugar controller works again.

Permanently remove from the diet all substandard junk fats and oils, as well as the processed and fast foods that contain them. When your blood sugar stabilizes, slowly introduce more healthy foods to the diet. Monitor your blood sugar levels to test the effect of these additional foods.

The goal of any effective program to reverse prediabetes and type 2 and possibly type 3 diabetes is to repair and restore the body's own blood sugar control mechanism. The malfunction of that eventually causes many of the debilitating symptoms.

Consume flax oils, fish oil, coconut, and olive oils. Add a broad number of minerals and vitamins, such as chromium and vitamins B12, D3, C, and E. Eat fiber-rich foods. Use only nontoxic sweetners like stevia. Maintain a balance of healthy fats, oils, lean proteins, and dense carbohydrates.

Some conditions, such as beginning retinopathy and peripheral neuropathy, can be reversed if permanent damage has not occurred. Kidney scarring probably can't be reversed. Excessive scarring of blood vessels in the eye cannot be reversed. Injections of certain steroids and Avastin (a former cancer drug that was used to kill tumors by destroying the blood vessels to the tumors) and laser surgery can correct a lot of vision problems, but eye vessel scarring will remain. Generally a lot of foot neuropathy can be reversed if the nerve damage is not too far gone.

# High-, Moderate-, and Low-Acid and Alkaline Foods and Beverages

## Neutral Substances

In the pH balance, neutral substances range from 6.5 to 7.5. Close to 7.5 is considered neutral.

Cancer cells cannot survive in a high-ph environment.

The definition of pH is the negative log of hydrogen in concentration in a water-based solution.

The definition of the power of hydrogen

> P came from the German word *poltzen*, meaning "power," and
> H is the element symbol for hydrogen.

Use the glycemic load-volume concept to balance pH.

pH is a logarithmic scale of 1 to 15, where 7.5 is considered to be neutral.

Sugar is a nonpolar compound, which doesn't dissolve into ions when put in water.

The negative ions of bases will tend to be healthier than the positive ions of acids.

NOTE: High-pH foods and beverages are not processed; they are raw.

## Alkaline Substances

pH      Food or Beverage

- baking soda

- raw broccoli, kale or mustard greens, lemon, and other green grasses

- loganberries, fresh mangos, pineapple, raspberries, artichokes, beets with their greens, raw celery, raw cucumber, endive, sweet potatoes, yams, unroasted diced pumpkin seeds, green and herbal teas, cilantro, parsley, and stevia plant

- blackberries, cantaloupe, honeydew (and most melons), fresh apricots, fresh dates, figs, grapefruit, grapes, kiwi, nectarines, fresh pears, papayas, passion fruit, raisins, alfalfa and other sprouted grains, carrots, fresh garlic, fresh ginger, green beans, most lettuces, onions and leeks, rutabagas, fresh sweet peas, ginger tea, cayenne, and cinnamon

## High-Acid Substances

- Regular table salt has a lower pH value. It is more acidic.

- apples, ripe bananas, fresh oranges, fresh peaches, bamboo shoots, beets without greens, chives, cooked brussels sprouts and broccoli, cooked pumpkin and eggplant, fresh tomato, turnip, parsnips and turnip greens, wild rice, and sesame seeds, almonds, natural unsweetened fruit juice, fish oil, unsweetened molasses, most fresh herbs and spices, vegetable sea salt, apple cider vinegar

- blueberries, fresh coconut, fresh cranberries and strawberries, bamboo shoots without greens, olives, cooked brussels sprouts and broccoli, cooked squash and eggplant, fresh corn, and okra, potatoes with skins, flaxseeds, chestnuts, unprocessed apple cider, grain coffee substitutes, flax and avocado oil, raw maple syrup, sea salt

pH     Food or Beverage

- egg yolks cooked soft, unsalted butter and margarine, bamboo shoots, beets without greens, brown and basmati rice, municipal tap water, canola, corn, and sunflower oil, barley malt syrup, and raw honey

- green bananas, cooked green peas, horseradish, kidney and pinto beans, cooked spinach, cooked whole eggs and egg whites, liver and other organ meats, processed cow and goat milk, processed dairy products (dairy products are slightly acidic), most cheeses, oats, buckwheat (herb), corn and rice, breads, cornmeal, buttered popcorn with no salt, sunflower seeds, wheat, rye rice crackers, whole grains, rice vinegar, soy sauce, carob, fructose, and pastries from honey and whole grain

- dates, figs and other dried fruits, cooked cranberries, and prunes, black-eyed peas, peeled potatoes, most pickles, cooked zucchini, salmon, tuna, and most other fish, oysters and most shellfish, plain yogurt, corn bread and tortillas, cream of wheat, most whole grain breads, popcorn with salt and butter, rye, wheat, and wheat germ, pistachios and pine nuts, kona coffee, soy, rice, and almond milk, salted butter, pumpkin- and grape-seed oil, processed maple syrup, sulfur and molasses, and hummus

- pomegranates, garbanzo beans, lima beans, chicken, turkey, duck, and goose, lamb and goat, venison and elk, processed cereals, white rice, semolina, wheat bran, white and wheat flour, Brazil nuts, walnuts, and pecans, sesame, safflower, and almond oil, reverse-osmosis filtered water, most bottled water and sport drinks, brown sugar, chocolate, custard with white sugar, sweetened yogurt, tapioca, ketchup, jarred mayonnaise, mustard, vanilla, and most pharmaceutical drugs

- most frozen and canned vegetables, swiss chard, navy beans, most wild game, cottage cheese, barley, oat bran, rice cakes, most wine, powdered or liquid stevia, balsam, cider vinegar, cigarettes, and iodized table salt

- beef and pork, mussels, squid, and other mollusks, goat cheese, white pasta, most beers, black teas, hard liquor, most coffee, sugar-added fruit juices, jams and jellies, pastries from white flour and sugar, white sugar, and most microwave foods and unsweetened cocoa (the preservatives are highly acidic)

- most legumes, snow peas, tomato sauce, veal, buttermilk, cream cheese, granola, white bread, flour tortillas, artificial sweeteners, and white vinegar

- canned tuna, lobster, ice cream, nuts, most roasted nuts, hazelnuts, carbonated soft drinks except colas, sugar-added grapefruit and orange juice, and cottonseed and palm oil

- bacon, sausages, processed chesses, colas (2.5 pH!), pudding, french fries and most other fried foods, sleep deprivation, and yeast

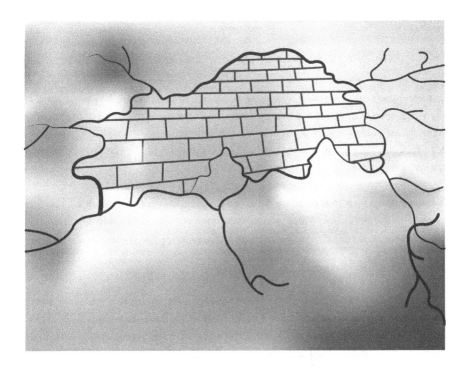

The Wall

# The BEST Syndrome

There are many contributing factors to the conditions that affect over 25 percent of the population of the United States with regard to insulin resistance, prediabetes, and type 1, type 2, and type 3 diabetes.

We use the acronym BEST to break down the various components of some but not all of the causes for these conditions.

- biological
- environmental (and economic)
- social
- technological

## Biological

Various biological factors certainly have an effect on the development and progress of various diseases such as heart disease, stroke, cancer, and the various types of diabetes, including possibly dementia and Alzheimer's disease (type 3 diabetes). Genetics are a big factor in getting a certain disease to start with. There are those who are extremely overweight and have never had high blood sugar (glucose) levels. Why would that be the case? Because they don't have the genetic marker for diabetes.

We have addressed markers in a separate chapter. Markers are genetic flags that alert us to the potential future development of a condition or disease.

## Environmental

**This category can be blamed for poor health in the general population more than anything else. We are daily bombarded by toxins that we touch, breathe, ingest, inhale, and absorb, along with plastics and Styrofoam-containing substances such as BPA. These substances can and do trigger insulin resistance in many people.**

More studies are coming out indicating that environmental exposure to chemicals such as ABS and other chemicals found in plastics and Styrofoam may indeed be responsible for obesity, insulin resistance, prediabetes, type 2 diabetes, and other various diseases. In a nutshell, our environment is *killing us*!

Even certain medications can affect our glucose (blood sugar) levels, such as the statin family of drugs used to lower bad (LDL) cholesterol. New studies are indicating possible connections between statins and dementia and Alzheimer's disease.

## Economic

Economics is partly to blame for our health problems. Living paycheck to paycheck, enduring stress at a job you don't like, and not being able to purchase the proper foods you need to eat for good health are a few examples of adverse effects caused by economics. The middle class of this country have become economic slaves who can't afford to pay for the necessary health care, prescriptions, and natural remedies to help make them well again. Against this background is a broken pharmaceutical and health care system that makes most people want to simply give up.

## Social

What can we say about our social environment? It's got a problem, that's what. We spend most of our lives subconsciously trying to be liked and accepted or trying to impress others with how smart, tough, and dazzling we are. We need to live for ourselves. That doesn't mean we don't help others. What we do to help our fellow humans is critical in our life's bucket list. But don't sell out to pressure. Don't be swayed by Fifth Avenue marketing. Be true to your principles.

We would suggest that you sit in front of your television one night and take note of all the commercials that you see; most of them are trying to sell you something to help counter what the other company sold you.

We have moved from a country that sold technology and training to the rest of the world to a consumption country. Our social fabric is based on consumption and heavy national and personal debt loads.

Don't blindly accept what everyone tells you. Ask questions—lots of questions. You have the right to defend yourself. Our hearts go out to those who can't afford decent housing, food, and medical attention.

Our society is highly technical but has become devoid of caring for others in need. Those who try to help have our gratitude.

## Technological

Here's an interesting question: Are we better off or worse off now than we were fifty years ago? Before you answer that question, think about it. Do you remember using your push mower to mow your yard? Remember the hand clippers you used to do the edging? Remember when we did not have remote controls for our televisions, stereos, and air conditioners? Do you remember riding a bicycle around town? Visiting with neighbors on the front porch and not having to arm your home security system is a thing of the past.

Now we are prisoners of our own modern marvels. We are overwhelmed with cell phone calls, texts, emails, and information at the touch of a button. These devices control us; we don't control them!

Now when we go see our doctors and medical professionals, they spend as much or more time entering our medical information into the health network computer system than examining us. It's not their fault. Driven by profit seeking, the medical insurance companies and the corporate medical providers are dictating how things are run, what you are covered for or not covered for, and some day whether you will live or die.

Don't let yourself be ignored or intimidated; stand up for your rights! Have family and friends help you if needed.

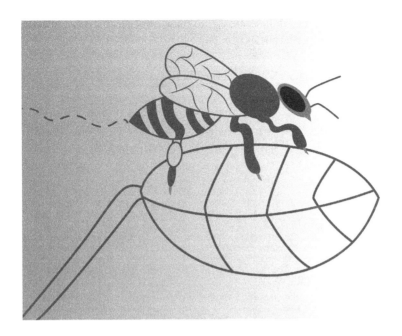

The Bee

# The Alkaline Diet

It's hard to imagine that many of our adverse medical conditions can stem from excess acid levels in our bodies. When we balance our chemical levels in our swimming pools, we strive for a 7.5 percent pH level, which is an even balance between the acid and alkaline levels. If the pH level is too high, you add chlorine (acid), and when the acid level is too high, you add soda ash (alkaline).

When you are preparing pasta sauce with heavy tomato paste, you can add a small amount of baking soda, which will make the tomato sauce mild; you can also add italian seasonings. You don't need to add sugar.

A lower-carbohydrate, gluten-free alkaline diet is becoming the diet regimen of choice. Recent studies are indicating that such a diet can stave off the onset of type 1 diabetes by as much as five years. We have included a chapter on the Mediterranean anti-inflammation diet (MAID), which incorporates these concepts. Along with that we have included a copy of the "Safe" House, a comprehensive food guide to good fats and carbohydrates and lean proteins.

It is possible to strike a balance between low carbohydrates and acidics.

You can have a low-carbohydrate, gluten-free, high-pH balanced diet. It's a question of balance. This balance will help you deter diabetes and its associated complications, such as heart disease, stroke risk, and even cancer.

# The Mediterranean Anti-Inflammation Diet (MAID)

The MAID is a combination of healthy complex carbohydrates (natural and dense), natural sugars, healthy fats (omega-3 fatty acids), and lean protein.

Diabetes and obesity cannot survive in the "Safe" House (see the illustration later in this chapter). You can venture out of the safe house occasionally. Diabetes and obesity will be out there waiting for you, but they won't be able to attack you when you're back in the safe house. If they follow you in there, they will wither and die.

Eat when you are hungry! Don't eat what you like. Like what you eat. It takes three weeks to develop a habit. Check with your doctor, diabetes educator, or dietitian regarding this program before starting it.

The MAID is both a Mediterranean diet and an anti-inflammation diet combined into one system. Timing is everything. It uses the concept of glycemic load, which goes beyond the glycemic index and takes into account the volume of the food along with the glycemic index (the speed at which foods convert to sugar in your bloodstream). You don't need complicated math. Just count from one to thirty processed carbohydrates between noon and eight in the evening. If you want to vary the time period somewhat, go ahead. Just watch your glucose readings for spikes (higher-than-normal glucose increases).

Carbohydrates and sugars consumed have to be either slowed or blocked from entering your bloodstream (absorbed), burned up as fuel, stored as fat, or left in your bloodstream, causing possible havoc if in too great a quantity. When we discuss the "Safe" House diagram, we will review spikers and stabilizers.

Chlorophyll comes from plants, just as protein comes from animals and nuts. We need both for good health. When you think of chlorophyll, think green. You want to eat green.

Our bodies build up toxins from our environment and from the foods we eat. Toxins and yeasts build up in our tissue cells, making them swollen and inflamed. The cells can then become insulin resistant. Chlorophyll helps to clean out those toxins and yeasts from our cells.

Spicy/hot foods tend to rev up our metabolism. The pepper family of foods contains capsaicin, which has various health benefits for prediabetes and type 2 diabetics. Capsaicin revs up the brown fat cells in our body, which regulate the energy burning in our bodies. Apparently capsaicin causes our white fat cells that haven't metabolized to become hybrid cells with mitochondria and in essence metabolize. Fat is released from the cells, and our bodies' enzymes remove it from our bodies. Neat trick, I'd say. Capsaicin prevents the release of insulin for about thirty minutes.

This is not a low-carbohydrate, low-fat, or high-protein diet. Everything is balanced. The MAID is healthy for the whole family.

# THE "SAFE" HOUSE

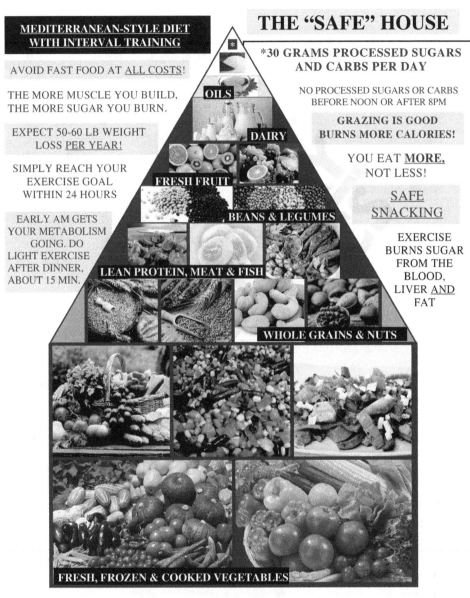

## MEDITERRANEAN-STYLE DIET WITH INTERVAL TRAINING

AVOID FAST FOOD AT ALL COSTS!

THE MORE MUSCLE YOU BUILD, THE MORE SUGAR YOU BURN.

EXPECT 50-60 LB WEIGHT LOSS PER YEAR!

SIMPLY REACH YOUR EXERCISE GOAL WITHIN 24 HOURS

EARLY AM GETS YOUR METABOLISM GOING. DO LIGHT EXERCISE AFTER DINNER, ABOUT 15 MIN.

*30 GRAMS PROCESSED SUGARS AND CARBS PER DAY

NO PROCESSED SUGARS OR CARBS BEFORE NOON OR AFTER 8PM

GRAZING IS GOOD BURNS MORE CALORIES!

YOU EAT MORE, NOT LESS!

SAFE SNACKING

EXERCISE BURNS SUGAR FROM THE BLOOD, LIVER AND FAT

OILS

DAIRY

FRESH FRUIT

BEANS & LEGUMES

LEAN PROTEIN, MEAT & FISH

WHOLE GRAINS & NUTS

FRESH, FROZEN & COOKED VEGETABLES

EAT GREEN (CHLOROPHYLL)

CAPSAICIN (METABOLIZE THE BROWN FAT CELLS AND THE WHITE FAT CELLS)

www.thediabetesslayershandbook.com Author ALAN D RAGUSO Copyright 2012 The "Safe House" illustrated byMegan Eaton

# Counting Processed Sugars and Carbohydrates

We could have titled this chapter "Carbohydrate Counting Kept Simple," "My Way," "Personalized Carbohydrate Counting," or even "Carbohydrate Counting with a Twist."

You might say, "A carb is a carb is a carb." Not so fast! Basically the three building blocks of food are proteins, fats, and carbohydrates. For now let's talk about carbs.

Some might say, "All carbohydrates are the same." That's not exactly the case. Some carbohydrates and certain sugars will be absorbed much faster than others. The sooner you understand this concept, the sooner you will be able to turn the tide against diabetes.

What about glycemic load? When I talk about sugar absorption, I am talking about sugar that goes into the bloodstream. This sugar is fine as long as it's burned up for fuel by the body's muscles or tissues. The sugar that is not burned up either will be stored in your fat cells, making you fatter, or simply remain floating around in your bloodstream, creating havoc with your health.

Get the monkey off your back! This refers to carbohydrate and sugar addiction. We eat natural and dense carbohydrates and natural sugars such as fructose, which is more slowly absorbed.

We take processed carbohydrates and subtract fiber and sugar alcohols to obtain a net carbohydrate number. Some experts recommend that you only subtract 50 percent of sugar alcohols from the carbohydrates. Some health experts don't worry about small numbers of either carbohydrates or fiber (three grams or less). We just subtract them all. If I have a net of two grams, three grams, and five grams from a total of three food items, we've had ten grams of carbohydrates.

**THE MAID** (Mediterranean Anti-Inflammation Diet) with LRIT (Low-Resistance Interval Training) … A Healthy Lifestyle-Transition Program

| The Problem | The Possible Cause | The Possible Response |
|---|---|---|
| Excess Weight | Consuming too many processed carbs & sugar; cell inflammation; lack of exercise; excess calorie intake; excess fat intake; leptin resistance; body releases cortisol due to stress; possible food allergies. | LRIT (lower it) capsaicin with dinner; chlorophyll (eat green); 7 hrs sleep; eat good fats; good carbs; lean protein; fiber & acidic foods (FAA); limit/avoid soy, wheat, & gluten; avoid fast foods!<br><br>Count calories; limit daily intake of processed carbs & sugars to 30 grams per day (consume them between noon & 8:00 p.m.). You can eat after 8:00 p.m. if you haven't exceeded your daily calorie intake.<br><br>Take 500 mg vitamin C each morning and evening. |
| Appetite Attacks | Leptin resistance; sugar; carb addiction; inactivity; the insulin yo-yo. | LRIT (lower it); reduce bad carbs; sugar; safe snacking; eat protein; good fats; keep mentally and physically active. |
| Higher than Normal Glucose/A1C | Excess intake of bad carbs & sugar; lack of exercise; cell inflammation (which interferes with insulin working effectively); the insulin yo-yo. | Add fiber & acidic foods to daily intake; LRIT (lower it).<br><br>Safe (planned) snacking (midmorning & midafternoon).<br><br>Eat lots of green vegetables (chlorophyll—eat green); this reduces cell inflammation.<br><br>Build muscle (muscle burns sugar); limit daily intake of processed carbs & sugars to 30 grams per day; take vitamin D. |

| Higher than Normal LDL & Triglycerides | Lack of exercise; excess intake of omega-6 fatty acids/saturated fats. | Increase fiber intake; take full daily recommended dosage of fish oil pills.<br><br>LRIT (lower it); consume capsaicin especially at dinner; avoid saturated fats. |
|---|---|---|
| Low HDL | Lack of exercise; low intake of omega-3 fatty acids. | LRIT (lower it); consume fish oil pills & small amount of olive & canola oils; black olives; walnuts; almonds; flaxseed; cold water fish (such as tuna). |
| High Blood Pressure | Lack of exercise; excess sodium intake; stress. | Reduce sodium intake; LRIT (lower it); 7 hrs sleep/night; reduce caffeine intake. |
| Joint & Tissue Pain | Food allergies; excess sugar absorption; lack of exercise. | LRIT (Lower it); reduce sugar intake; eat fiber & acidics. |

**Note:** LRIT (lower it) and capsaicin will keep your metabolism going virtually twenty-four hours per day! Capsaicin delays the release of insulin by thirty minutes. Insulin creates an appetite surge; also, insulin may make you gain weight. Read your food labels! Metabolism is the conversion of food into living material and into energy.

## The Three Ps and the Four Bs

If it's packaged, it's probably processed.
Ban it, burn it, block it (using the) back door—fiber and acidic.

Lettuce with vinegar and citrus helps block the absorption
of sugar; eat your salad *before* your main meal.

# Minerals, Vitamins, and Micronutrients

Micronutrients are involved in carbohydrate metabolism, glucose metabolism, insulin release, and insulin sensitivity.

Trace elements and water-soluble vitamin losses (vitamin D) are increased during uncontrolled hyperglycemia and glycosuria, a condition characterized by an excess of sugar in the urine, typically associated with diabetes and kidney disease.

Serum or tissue content of copper, manganese, iron, and selenium can be higher in people without DM (diabetes mellitus).

Serum vitamin C, B vitamins, and vitamin D are often lower in individuals with DM, while levels of vitamins A and E have been reported to be normal or higher.

Vitamin receptors (VDRs) are found in all insulin-responsive tissues, as well as in pancreatic beta cells. They interfere with normal metabolism. Vitamin D suppresses macrophage migration. VDRs are found on many cells. Vitamin D plays a role in decreasing the inflammatory response in inflammatory pathways.

## Vitamin D

Vitamin D appears to play a role in cholesterol metabolism.

Many observational studies have linked vitamin D deficiency to an increased risk of type 2 diabetes mellitus (T2 DM).

Epidemiological studies show correlations between low serum vitamin D concentrations and increased insulin resistance and impaired beta cell function.

An NHANES study showed an inverse correlation between serum 25 (OH) D concentrations and the incidence of T2 DM.

2015 diabetes world summit advice on which supplements help with blood sugar.

Vitamin D supplementation given in early childhood has been found to decrease type 1 diabetes. Serum vitamin D is inversely correlated with body fat. Is the low vitamin D or obesity increasing the risk of type 2 diabetes?

One would be advised to keep higher levels of vitamin D and maintain a healthy body weight. Don't use BMI (body mass index)—use our body density composition.

Vitamin D deficiency and high serum levels of vitamin D also affect serum calcium levels, and calcium is a critical ion in insulin secretion and action. Keeping calcium levels normal may result in normal glucose tolerance and beta cell function. Vitamin D supplements may reduce the risk of developing insulin resistance, prediabetes, and type 2 diabetes.

Fifty thousand units of vitamin D3 daily for eight weeks reduced insulin resistance within eight weeks in a group study of one hundred patients. Ten minutes of midday sunlight on the arms and legs provides ten thousand units of vitamin D per day.

Raspberries are high in vitamin B12. Low serum B12 and foliate (vitamin B9) levels have been linked to increased oxidative stress markers in people living with diabetes. People living with diabetes who have low levels of B12 are more likely to have peripheral (feet and hands) neuropathy compared to people who do not have low B12 levels.

Thirty-four million Americans over sixty-five years of age have prediabetes. There is a high number of patients with insulin resistance, prediabetes, and type 1 and type 2 diabetes with vitamin B12 deficiencies; foliate works with B12. If too much vitamin B is taken, the body will eliminate it like vitamin C. Folic acid is synthetic (made in a lab) and can build up too high in the body. Persons with the MHHFR gene must not take folic acid as a supplement to food or in vitamins. Folic acid foods include dark leafy greens, asparagus, avocado, cauliflower, seeds, and nuts, as well as beets. Avoid grain products "fortified with folic acid."

## Vitamin C

Vitamin C is found in foods like broccoli. People with diabetes tend to have lower blood levels of vitamin C than those with no diabetes. Some experts believe that low serum vitamin C levels contribute to the depressed immune function, compromised wound healing ability, and reduced blood vessel integrity that are seen in diabetes.

Chronic low-grade inflammation resulting from oxidative stress has been associated with insulin resistance.

Antioxidants may reduce the level of protein glycation and DNA damage caused by hyperglycemias.

Vitamin C is an antioxidant and has been found to play a role in both iron absorption and wound healing. It's best to get your vitamin C from daily dietary intake. High doses can cause renal stones.

Foods with vitamin C include bell peppers, kale, broccoli, cauliflower, papayas, oranges, strawberries, and parsley.

## Zinc

Zinc appears to help reduce insulin resistance. Type 2 diabetics can experience better glucose control with zinc supplements.

You can find zinc in seafood, beef and lamb, pork, chicken, cashews, pumpkin seeds, spinach, mushrooms, beans, and cocoa powder.

## Magnesium

Magnesium is a cofactor of various enzymes in carbohydrate oxidation, and it plays an important role in the glucose-transporting mechanism of the cell membrane.

Magnesium is involved in insulin secretion, binding, and activity. A health study conducted by nurses showed an association between greater magnesium intake and lower incidence of type 2 diabetes.

Observational studies have shown hypomagnesemia occurs more frequently in patients with type 2 diabetes, especially those with poor glycemic control. Magnesium requirements can be met through food intake.

High doses of magnesium supplements often result in diarrhea, which can be accompanied by nausea and abdominal cramping.

Foods with magnesium include spinach, nuts and seeds, almonds, cashews, peanut butter, soymilk, beans and lentils, fish, baked potatoes, yogurt, bananas and avocados, and zinc soft gels.

## Cinnamon

Studies indicate cinnamon helps reduce insulin resistance. A word of caution: cinnamon oil contains coumarone, a blood thinner.

## Chocolate

Consuming 200 mg of flavonols from chocolate has been shown to improve blood flow. There is promising evidence that flavonols can lower blood pressure and improve brain function.

Flavonols from chocolate can come from cocoa powder, baking chocolate, semisweet chocolate chips, dark chocolate, chocolate syrup, and milk chocolate. Cocoa that is processed with alkali, or dutch processed, contains almost no flavonols.

## Summary

As you have probably noticed, our food list (pgs. 70-73) contains items that are both low in processed carbohydrates and sugars and are gluten-free. If patients use the system correctly, it's almost impossible to fail. Slowing and blocking carbohydrates from being absorbed, plus burning and neutralizing sugars and cranking the metabolism to 24-7, is a deadly one-two punch to both obesity and diabetes. An increased intake of chlorophyll (eating green) helps to greatly reduce insulin resistance by getting the cells to reduce cell inflammation and swelling. Add low-resistance interval training, and you should start feeling better immediately.

It is our sincerest hope that you review our first book, *The Diabetes Slayer's Handbook: Preventing or Reversing Prediabetes and Type 2 Diabetes*. In this book, we have built on the concepts of that book and gone out much further in our delivery of ideas and effective approaches to fight the deadly disease called diabetes.

You have probably noticed our food charts are full of items that are anti-inflammatory; low in poor-quality preservatives, processed carbohydrates, and sugars; and are gluten-free. By slowing and blocking the carbohydrates being absorbed in your bloodstream and burning and neutralizing sugars and increasing your metabolic rate, you create an effective opposition to insulin resistance, prediabetes, and type 2 and type 3 diabetes. Lower carbohydrate intake will help a lot to start with. An increased intake of chlorophyll (eating green) helps to greatly reduce insulin resistance by reducing cell inflammation and swelling. Add low-resistance interval training, along with weight training and resistance training, and you should start seeing results and feeling better immediately.

Type 3 diabetes is a term you won't hear much right now, but in the years to come, you will hear about it. If you take the right steps now, you may be able to prevent or at least delay this new form of diabetes, dementia and Alzheimer's disease.

If you are taking metformin, are over sixty years old, or are a vegan, consider taking a daily vitamin B12 supplement. Get your serum B12 and vitamin D levels checked at least once a year. If either level is low, talk to your doctor about taking a supplement. The dose depends on the severity of the deficiency; avoid megadoses of all supplements except vitamin D and vitamin B12.

Eat a variety of unprocessed foods, including vegetables, nuts, and seeds. Refer to the "Safe" House illustration and the Mediterranean anti-inflammation diet (MAID).

Diet drinks trigger the release of dopamine.

Eat natural foods, and avoid processed foods and drinks.

Keep active and move around. For every thirty minutes of sitting, move around for two minutes.

Do you want to improve your health and live a better, longer life? You have to pay for the bus ride.

If you want to find out how to get blood tests to find out where you are in terms of dietary supplements, consult your medical caregiver.

## Labs to Ask For

- CMP: Comprehensive Metabolic Profile: magnesium, potassium, calcium, and sodium. This tells what is in the blood. These four electrolytes help maintain our healthy hearts beating with chemical stimulation.
- RBC (Red Blood Cell) labs for magnesium and potassium to tell what is actually in the cells.
- Homocysteine and fasting insulin.
- MTHFR: Tells how much B12 is actually getting to the cells. It tells if your body processes B12, D3, and T3 properly, and it shows your genetic risk for disease.
- If you have the MTHFR, also get tested for T3, D3, and D1.25.
- D3.
- Sex hormones (which cause insulin resistance). Women should be tested for estradiol, progesterone, DHEA, and free testosterone. Men should have the same tests and add to the above labs dihydrotestosterone.
- Ferritin, which tells how much iron you have in your cells, which affects insulin resistance.
- Folic acid.
- Chromium.
- Zinc.

## Supplement Doses for Insulin Resistance

- Cinnamon, 1/2–1 tsp/day. Caution: cinnamon can thin your blood. Ask your doctor before you begin using it.
- Magnesium: Always take with calcium. Magnesium causes the body to lose calcium; ask your doctors about a daily dose of 500 mg, 1000 calcium, and 15 zinc. Zinc: 50 mg/day.
- Vitamin C: RDA is 75–2000/day.
- B12: Methyl B12 lozenges/liquid 5000 in 1–4 lozenges/day (metformin, MTHFR) (if you have) (if you are over sixty).
- Chromium: Normal dosage 200–600 iu. Insulin resistance dose, 1,000 iu.
- Chocolate: 200 mg flavonols/day for insulin resistance.

Blood Sugar Goals

- Normal Fasting: under 85 mg/dl
- Diabetes: under 110 mg/dl
- Normal two hours postmeal: under 120 mg/dl
- Diabetes two hours postmeal: under 140 mg/dl
- Diabetes and on insulin: under 160 mg/dl postmeal

# Low-Carbohydrate Diets

There have been a number of research articles out recently indicating that a very low-carbohydrate diet can help prevent or even reverse diabetes. Some of these diets have some promise of accomplishing just what they say they can do. There are a few medical doctors who suggest a daily *total* intake of only twenty grams of carbohydrates is plenty for a person to stay healthy. Indeed, it can be argued that we don't need *any* carbohydrates for our brain function and overall general health. Our bodies will convert some protein eventually into carbohydrates.

Once again, a word of caution: don't embark on *any type* of weight-loss program before seeking competent medical advice. Dropping to a total intake of only twenty grams of carbohydrates per day may not be possible to sustain over a long period of time. Whatever you do to stabilize your blood sugar *must be sustainable*.

Here are foods for a low-carbohydrate diet that are rich in vitamins, minerals, and nutrients.

Vitamin A: liver, cod liver oil, broccoli, butter, kale, spinach, collard greens, some cheeses, and eggs

Vitamin B1: pork, sunflower seeds, asparagus, kale, cauliflower, liver, and eggs

Vitamin B2: asparagus, cottage cheese, meat, eggs, fish, and green beans

Vitamin B3: liver, heart, kidney, chicken, beef, fish (tuna, salmon), eggs, avocados, leafy vegetables, broccoli, asparagus, nuts, and mushrooms

Vitamin B5: meats, broccoli, and avocados

Vitamin B6: meats and nuts

Vitamin B7: egg yolk, liver, and some vegetables

Vitamin B9 (a.k.a. folate or acid folic): liver, sunflower seeds, avocado, broccoli, dark leafy greens, asparagus, nuts, and cauliflower

Vitamin B12: fish, shellfish, meat, poultry, eggs, and dairy products

Vitamin C: peppers, liver, kale, broccoli, cauliflower, and strawberries

Vitamin D: produced in the skin after exposure to ultraviolet B light from the sun or artificial sources; also found in fatty fish, eggs, beef liver, and mushrooms

Vitamin E: almonds, avocado, eggs, and leafy green vegetables

Vitamin K: leafy green vegetables, avocado, brussels sprouts, and parsley

Omega-3s: salmon, tuna, halibut, oysters, avocado, spinach, kale, and walnuts

Calcium: almond milk, cheeses, spinach, broccoli, clams, and beef

Iron: clams, oysters, and organ meats like liver; also spinach

Zinc: seafood like oysters are also zinc rich, along with spinach, cashews, and dark chocolate.

Chromium: processed meats, green beans, romaine lettuce, broccoli, nuts, and egg yolk

Magnesium: dark leafy greens, nuts, seeds, fish, avocados, and dark chocolate

Potassium: almonds, beef, blackberries, broccoli, brussels sprouts, clams, salmon, tuna, turkey, avocado, spinach, kale, and beef

Phosphorus: cheese, nuts, veal, mushrooms, scallops, sardines, salmon, and shrimp

Sodium: salt, cured meat, some cheeses, pickles

Fluorine: pickles, spinach, asparagus, avocados, brussels sprouts, cauliflower, cucumber, green leafy vegetables, nuts (especially almonds), seafood, and tinned fish

Pantothenic acid: animal liver and kidney, fish, shellfish, pork, chicken, egg yolk, mushrooms, avocados, and broccoli

Manganese: seafood, leafy greens, and hazelnuts

Copper: leafy greens, including turnip greens, spinach, swiss chard, kale and mustard greens, walnuts, oysters and other shellfish, and organ meats (kidneys, liver)

Selenium: Brazil nuts, seafood, fish, pork, beef, lamb, chicken, turkey, and mushrooms

Even if you don't eat veggies (which you should because they are delicious), you can still get a lot of vitamins and nutrients.

3 oz. (85g) of beef contain: calcium 1%, iron 12%, vitamin D 1%, vitamin B6 15%, vitamin B12 36%, and magnesium 4%

1 large egg contains: vitamin A 5%, calcium 2%, iron 3%, vitamin D 11%, vitamin B6 5%, vitamin B12 10%, and magnesium 1%

1 oz. (28g) cheddar cheese contains: vitamin A 5%, calcium 20%, iron 1%, vitamin D 1%, vitamin B12 3%, and magnesium 2%

So no worries about your nutrients. You probably are getting enough.

# Glycemic Load

Glycemic load takes into account the quality of the glycemic index number in addition to the quantity of a food. It is a much more accurate scale than simply the glycemic index. Glycemic load considers the quality of the carbohydrates (how quickly one gram converts to sugar in the bloodstream) as well as the quantity of the carbohydrate (how many grams or ounces are consumed).

We use glycemic load counting when we count carbohydrates and balance our food intake. Some foods rated high in carbohydrates on the glycemic index actually fall into the moderate rating in the glycemic load index. You can eat some foods high in carbohydrates in smaller amounts and some foods lower in carbohydrates in higher amounts and have virtually the same net effect on blood glucose levels.

Please refer to our chapter "The Three States of Carbohydrates" when considering glycemic load. The speed at which a carbohydrate converts to blood glucose is vitally important, just as is the carbohydrate density of the food item.

Some foods will appear higher on the glycemic index than they will on the glycemic load index. For instance, strawberries and watermelon will appear to be higher in blood sugar conversion but you have to eat a lot of either one of these two fruits to get a significant blood glucose increase.

So we want to take into account not just the carbohydrate with respect to the glycemic index (quality) but the volume of that food (quantity) and the speed (rate of glucose absorption) of the food item in question.

Some experts will tell you that viewing carbohydrates this way is not necessary. However, if you can avoid glucose bumps and spikes, we feel you can go a long way in preventing ongoing vessel damage to your body and avoiding complications.

# Maintaining Low Glucose Levels

Is maintaining low glucose levels a good strategy for preventing lots of complications, such as eye, kidney, and heart problems, as well as dementia and Alzheimer's disease?

What have you got to lose?

Many people who are prediabetics have complications.

Medical professionals are now starting to suggest having an A1C level of 6.5 instead of 7.0. The day may come that they recommend having an A1C level of 6.0 or lower. Talk to your doctor for their opinion. Remember your doctor has the final say about treating your medical conditions. If you retain a doctor, then trust your doctor in the final analysis.

Study the A1C/eAG conversion chart below. "You can't know where you're going if you don't know where you are."

## A1C to eAG Conversion Chart

This table shows the relationship between A1C and eAG, estimated average glucose.

| A1C% | eAG mg/dl |
| --- | --- |
| 5 | 97 |
| 5.5 | 111 |
| 6 | 126 |
| 6.5 | 140 |
| 7 | 154 |
| 7.5 | 169 |
| 8 | 183 |
| 8.5 | 197 |
| 9 | 212 |
| 9.5 | 226 |
| 10 | 240 |
| 10.5 | 255 |
| 11 | 269 |

Three points on your glucose monitor db/per liter equals one-tenth of a percentage point on your A1C level. If our monitor were to register 111, we know the A1C equivalent is 5.5.

If you had two separate glucose readings of 120 and 140, you would add those together and divide by 2, which gives you an average of 130, which is about a 6.2 A1C equivalent.

# The Four Bs

Slowing or blocking the absorption of sugar into your bloodstream can be accomplished by using the four Bs.

## Ban It

If you don't eat a high-carbohydrate or sugar item to start with, there's no way that sugar will get into your system.

## Burn It

A simple way to eliminate blood sugar (glucose) is to burn it up using exercise. I'm not talking about grinding yourself into the ground with exhausting workouts. You can burn sugar with simple low-resistance exercise and by simply moving around.

## Block It

This technique has been used for weight loss, but guess what? It works to block, slow down, or even stop the absorption of sugar into your bloodstream, using the back door.

## Back Door

To use the back door, you use a one-two punch of fiber and acidics (FAA). First is fiber. Fiber slows and even blocks sugar absorption. Second is acidics, such as plain vinegars and citrus juices (lime, lemon, and grapefruit juices), which *neutralize sugar*! Stick to plain, unseasoned vinegars and vinaigrettes. The seasoned ones generally have a number of carbohydrates in them and may be higher in calories.

# The Three Ps

How do you determine if a food product is refined or processed? If it's *packaged*, it's probably processed. That means it's suspect. You have to read the label to see what is contained in foods.

Reading food labels is one of the most important things you can do. I think it's every bit as important as exercise.

Have you ever had someone give you something to taste and they said, "Go ahead and try it; it's *good* for you"?

Never taste something that is mysteriously vague. If you can't see an ingredient label for the food product, don't eat it! Would you swallow mysterious unmarked pills? Of course you wouldn't.

Learn to understand what you're eating. It will empower you to control your health destiny.

# Stocking Your Food Arsenal

Learn to like what you eat instead of eating what you like. I read a story several years ago about a man who went overseas for several years. At first he did not like the food in the country he went to, but then he realized it was very healthy and got used to eating it. He had learned to like what he ate. When he returned to the United States, he was appalled at the poor quality of food here and continued to eat the foods that he had eaten when he was overseas. Instead of eating what we like, we need to learn to like what we eat. It takes three weeks to develop a habit. Once you develop a taste for certain healthy foods, you will learn to enjoy them. Later when you taste some of the foods you were previously eating that were unhealthy, you will find that they no longer taste good to you. Your taste buds can be reprogrammed within a short amount of time to adapt to the new foods you are eating.

Processed foods and sugars are designed for fast preparation and quick eating. In order for the foods to be prepared quickly, a key ingredient is basically removed. That ingredient is dietary fiber. Fiber comes in a water-soluble form and an insoluble form. These fibers are one of your safeguards to slowing dramatically the absorption of sugars into your bloodstream. Remove the fiber, and one of your body's safety nets is removed.

There are many great-tasting foods that have a very low amount of digestible carbohydrates and sugars. Some foods are actually free of tangible carbohydrates and sugars.

When it comes to both losing weight and stabilizing your blood sugars, these are the kinds of foods you want to be eating, along with doing light to moderate exercise.

Calories Saved

You can save a lot of calories by simply making small changes in what you eat.

Spray oils—150 calories
Cheese sprinkles—150 calories
Smart bread—150 calories
Reduce coatings and breading—350 calories
One 1000–1200 mg fish oil pill taken in the evening—400 calories (It also raises your HDL like crazy!)
One medium 60-calorie egg in the morning—400 calories because of increased metabolic burn
Replace some of your salad dressings with plain vinegars and citrus juices. It's okay to put a packet of no-calorie sweetener made with sucralose on your salad if you want it sweeter—250 "zero everything" raspberry vinaigrette.
Light biking/walking—150 calories
Eliminate corn and potatoes—200 calories
Chicken or beef broth in the evening helps in weight reduction. Cut the portion size in half to reduce the sodium level. This product is also available in low sodium.
Drink 25 ounces of green tea per day to aid in weight reduction.
You can easily reduce your daily calorie intake by 2,000 calories without feeling deprived!

There's an arsenal of delicious foods available that you can use that are inexpensive everyday items right in your grocery store.

This list is only a small portion of what's available out there.

Vitamins B1, B12, and biotin increase the metabolism, and this combination doesn't upset your stomach like the B complex vitamins; vitamin D3 helps reduce glucose levels.

You may want to eat peeled apples. Half the sugars and carbohydrates are in the peeling. However, the apple peel is rich in phytochemicals. You can research this concept and decide whether or not to peel your apple.

Sugar-free chocolate and caramel toppings go with virtually zero everything. There's sugar-free gelatin and puddings, sugar-free bread and butter pickles, and sugar-free coffee flavorings in caramel, chocolate, raspberry, and hazelnut.

Fresh cooked vegetables are great; sometimes frozen ones are okay.

Use no-calorie sweetener, made with sucralose, not aspartame.

Use liquid butter spray (made from xanthan and guar gums).

Light mayonnaise comes from either canola or olive oil.

Sea salt has half the sodium, and the iodine is not depleted.

Red pepper hot sauces are good, as are precooked egg patties (or freshly cooked eggs).

Green relish has no sugar.

Negative-calorie foods take more calories to process than are contained in them and include lettuce, onions, mushrooms, and so on.

# Low—Glycemic Load Foods

The following is a partial list of low glycemic load foods:

turkey and fish products
sugar-free jams
lightly salted rice cakes
fudge pops, no sugar added
no-sugar-added fruit bars
unsweetened vanilla almond milk—your milk substitute
tuna—a cold water fish
reduced-sugar ketchup
carbohydrate-friendly pasta—only 5 grams of carbohydrates instead of 42
fresh fruits
pearl barley
brown rice
walnuts, almonds, and sunflower kernels
black olives
long cooking oats
*turmeric
*curry
*cinnamon
*mint
*ginger

*These spices increase metabolism.

Sugar alcohols commonly found in foods are sorbitol, mannitol, xylitol, isomalt, and hydrogenated starch hydrolysates; these sugars are derived from vegetation and are very slow to be sent into the bloodstream.

# Resistance Training and Weight Training to Reduce Insulin Resistance

Before we start this chapter, once again we must point out that before you start any exercise program or change your current one, you should consult your doctor. Even though many exercises that you do may seem relatively simple, seek out advice from professional physical trainers and other medical professionals and exercise counselors. You do not want to injure yourself. It's counterproductive, and it hurts!

Many recent studies and articles indicate that physical exercise will help in the absorption of blood sugar into the body's muscles. Since our muscles are the engines that burn fuel, it would make sense that exercising those muscles will reduce the excess sugar levels in our blood.

Remember our chapter on the four Bs. There are only so many ways to handle the sugar energy that we derive from food. Burning it is one way. The chapter preceding this one discussed low-resistance interval training (lower it). Resistance training and weight training rely on a given number of repetitions of a certain exercise (reps) to form a total number of reps (a set). For example, you may do ten reps (repetitions) of lifting barbells to form one set. As you rotate through various sets of exercises, you may find that you complete a total of three sets of lifting barbells.

Get professional advice about your personal training plan.

Resistance training uses your own body in a sense to create a resistance against the force you apply with a device as simple as a piece of elastic tubing, an exercise ball, or even a chair. This type of exercise will be slow and methodical. Like the low-resistance interval training, "fast and hard" is not the name of the game. Doing resistance training slowly will get very good results without serious risk of injury. Do be careful with elastic bands. Have them double wrapped around your hand. You do not want a band to slap you in the face!

You will do a certain number of reps and sets. Be patient; you will get results. Remember the NASA astronauts used resistance training for virtually the past sixty years!

Weight training employs either free weights (Olympic-style weights) or various types of commercial gym devices, such as professional training circuit equipment you would find at a professional gym. We recommend that you do such exercises at a facility with professional full-time trainers. You will be coached on proper techniques to maximize results and avoid injuries.

You should see your glucose levels start to drop after about two weeks. Monitor your progress. Once again, these exercises will be done in repetitions (reps) and sets.

Balance training consists of exercises to help maintain your equilibrium and balancing skills, which improves your agility and may even help you prevent serious falls or accidents. Exercise may help in your mental sharpness also, making you more focused and alert.

# Six Key Hormones You Should Know About

There are six important hormones you should know about.

- *Cortisol* is released by stress; it can be combated with omega-3 fatty acids, vitamin C, and low-resistance interval training (LRIT).

- *Ghrelin*'s release triggers appetite; counter its release with fiber, lean protein, and good-fat consumption.

- *Leptin* is a hormone released from the fat cells to signal the brain that energy has been sent to the cells; the brain may be leptin resistant and not recognize the signals. Use LRIT exercise to get the brain to start receiving the "all's full" signal.

- *Insulin* should only be released in small amounts when needed and not wasted; it triggers appetite and weight gain. Capsaicin delays the release of insulin by thirty minutes; you flip off the appetite (not hunger) switch by controlling the release of ghrelin, insulin, and cortisol and improving the brain reception of leptin signals.

  Insulin is produced by beta cells in the pancreas. Beta cells can degenerate and become depleted over time. Moderate exercise can possibly regenerate or increase their numbers. Scientific studies indicate this. You could make your pancreas healthier. *What a thought!*

- *Glucagon* has the opposite effect from insulin. It raises glucose levels.

Produced by the alpha cells in the pancreas. Studies indicate that when beta cells are severely depleted, alpha cells can take over their function! Also, there are other stress hormones released early in the morning to get our system going for the day. These hormones interfere with insulin.

- *Growth hormone (GH)*, also known as *Somatotropine* (or as *human growth hormone* [hGH or HGH] in its human form), is a peptide hormone that stimulates growth, cell reproduction, and cell regeneration in humans and other animals. When combined with cortisol, these two hormones can create insulin resistance in the very early hours of the morning.

# Timing Is Everything

What you need to understand about prediabetes and type 2 diabetes is that so many of your glucose highs and lows are a result of imbalanced food combinations and poor timing.

You need to develop a sense of "plate balance." That means that your meals need to have good balanced portions of healthy fats containing omega-3 fatty acids, lean protein, and natural dense (complex) carbohydrates. Your portions need to be measured and controlled. Dense, complex carbohydrates can be eaten in sizable quantities. We limit my consumption of processed carbohydrates and sugars to only thirty grams per day; we round out the rest of my carbohydrates (120–140) per day with the natural dense carbohydrates.

We exercise daily. My weapon of choice is an exercise bike. Just remember the best exercise for you is the one that you like and will stay with. Day after day, week after week, month after month, and year after year, you will continue to get healthier.

Work to reduce your postmeal glucose levels after your evening meal. This offsets your morning readings.

If your evening dinner contains a sensible amount of processed sugars and carbohydrates and your bedtime snacks consist of lean proteins and good fats and you've maintained moderate body mobility, you should see surprisingly good glucose readings the next morning.

We eat constantly during the day and even into the evening. Grazing is good. Your metabolism has to work at burning up the food you're eating; therefore, your metabolism is elevated.

It's not *how much* you eat but *what* you eat that counts.

You should add foods rich in chlorophyll to your daily diet. You eat these *in addition* to your normal food intake.

You should eat *more* food, not *less*!

Don't try to starve yourself. That's a recipe (no pun intended) for disaster!

We use food products that are diabetic friendly.

Eat apples; they help to stabilize glucose levels.
Sugar-free chocolate and caramel toppings top virtually zero everything.
sugar-free gelatin and puddings
sugar-free bread and butter pickles
sugar-free coffee flavorings: caramel, chocolate, raspberry, and hazelnut
Fresh cooked vegetables; sometimes frozen are okay.
no-calorie sweetener (made with sucralose)
liquid butter spray (xanthan and guar gums)
light mayonnaise (either canola or olive oil)
sea salt (half the sodium, and the iodine is not depleted)
red pepper hot sauces
precooked egg patties
green relish, no sugar
negative-calorie foods: lettuce, onions, mushrooms, and so on

## Low- to Moderate-Glycemic Load Foods

turkey and fish products
sugar-free jams
lightly salted rice cakes
fudge pops, no sugar added
no-sugar-added fruit bars
unsweetened vanilla almond milk—your milk substitute
tuna—cold water fish
reduced sugar ketchup
carbohydrate-friendly pasta—only 5 grams of carbohydrates instead of 42
fresh fruits
pearl barley
brown rice
walnuts, almonds, and sunflower kernels
black olives
long cooking oats
*turmeric
*curry
*cinnamon

*mint
*ginger

*These spices increase metabolism.

Prepare raw and cooked vegetables, snacks, and entrees ahead of time. Refrigerate or freeze them. We're fortunate to have so many great-tasting food substitutes to use that are extremely low in refined carbohydrates and sugars.

Sucralose will work better than aspartame for cooking because it doesn't break down from the heat of cooking.

# Genetics and Biomarkers

More and more compelling information is emerging that connects our family medical history, genetics, and environmental influences such as chemicals and toxins, combined with inflammation and stress.

Based on a review of medical journals and textbooks, the following family and relationships to us by family member(s) statistically affect our risk of diabetes as listed:

Type 1 Diabetes

Type 2 Diabetes

| Relative with Diabetes | Your Estimated Risk | Relative with Diabetes | Your Estimated Risk |
|---|---|---|---|
| Mother | 1–5% | Mother | 5–20% |
| Father | 5–15% | Father | 15–20% |
| Both Parents | 1–25% | Both Parents | 25–50% |
| Brother/Sister | 5–10% | Brother/Sister | 25–50% |
| Identical Twin | 25–50% | Identical Twin | 60–75% |

The medical definition of a *marker* is "a diagnostic indication for presence of a disease." It is something that identifies or that is used to identify. "Biomarkers" are physiological substances that may indicate disease when present in abnormal amounts in serum, as that caused by a malignancy.

There are many types of markers, some of which are *genetic markers*. In addition, there are bone markers, cardiac markers, pan B cell markers, pan T cell markers, and tumor markers, to name some but not all markers.

Testing markers include antibodies and C peptide.

## The MTHFR Gene

There is an inexpensive lab test that tests the level of methylfolate (vitamin B9), which prevents damage to blood vessels and helps to combat cognitive memory loss (CML).

There are at least forty mutations of the MTHFR gene that have been identified in people with homocystinuria, a disorder in which the body is unable to process certain amino acids properly.

Diabetics would want to get their homocysteine levels checked.

The MTHFR gene is needed for the multistep process that converts amino acid homocysteine to another amino acid, methionine.

The body uses methionine to proteins and other important compounds.

Variations in the methyl cycle can cause high homocysteine levels, possibly leading to vascular disease, dementia, Alzheimer's disease, and certain types of colon cancer.

# Convergence

The term *convergence* refers to the repetition of successful concepts that seem to work well over and over through time.

For example, in biology hinged appendages seem to be successful for many species for millions of years. If your body cannot convert carbohydrates to sugar and then into energy, would it not make sense to eat fewer carbohydrates and balance them with lean proteins and good fats?

Much about dealing with diabetes boils down to common sense. Yes, we have to eat, but we have to avoid foods that are bad for us.

# The Connection of Low pH Levels to Inflammation, Insulin Resistance, and Type 2 and Type 3 Diabetes

Once you gain understanding of the chain of conditions that finally lead to type 3 diabetes (some forms of dementia and Alzheimer's disease), you will be both fascinated and alarmed about the causes and implications. We all age, and with age our risks of debilitation and life-threatening diseases increase naturally.

There was a cartoon once with the young daughter looking at her mother in a restaurant and stating, "I don't have to watch what I eat. I'm eighteen years old!"

We run the risk of our future health failing due to causes that we and even our medical caregivers can't see coming. But you can beat them.

It has been said that conventional medical practice is ten years behind the science. We have to be careful that we do not jump on every new medical "breakthrough" or "cure" that comes along. There are thousands of books promoting diabetes "cures." We are here to say and stand by our statement that there is not a "cure" for type 1 or type 2 diabetes at this time. We can hope that someday cures will be developed for those conditions. Some conditions can be reversed, which is a tremendous health victory, but it's not a permanent cure. The conditions can come back with a vengeance. We believe you can do better than just control these conditions.

Getting back to the basics of eating fresh foods that have not been refined or processed is essential to getting your body balanced and operating at its peak without drugs or invasive procedures. A high-pH or alkaline diet is the opposite of a high-acid diet, and natural foods and beverages tend to be high in alkaline or low in acid. Keep in mind that acidic foods such as lemon, lime, and grapefruit juices change to an alkaline (nonacid) state when consumed. When we talk about healthy acidic foods and beverages, this is what we refer to.

Continued high acidic levels in the body can eventually lead to a host of adverse conditions. Inflammation is a cause for many illnesses and diseases. It can be argued that some types of heart disease, for instance, are more influenced by inflammation than things such as cholesterol levels.

Insulin resistance is often overlooked as a potential medical problem. We consider insulin resistance as a precursor to prediabetes. Just as prediabetes was not taken seriously as a warning flag for future type 2 diabetes, insulin resistance is not viewed seriously as a medical threat in many cases.

Take our word for it. It is a serious medical threat.

Not all people who have developed cognitive memory loss, dementia, and Alzheimer's disease had diagnosed diabetes. The medical community has for some time not worried about elderly patients having elevated glucose (blood sugar) levels because of their age. Yet this condition can eventually lead to the death of key brain cells that affect memory and other cognitive (reasoning) skills. You do not have to necessarily go through all the stages of poor pH control, insulin resistance, prediabetes, and type 2 diabetes to develop type 3 diabetes (dementia and Alzheimer's disease). Your odds of developing dementia or Alzheimer's disease are four times greater if you are a type 2 diabetic.

In the year 2000 there was no diagnosis of prediabetes. We all need to recognize that these various conditions we have pointed out are warning flags, which we need to heed before years down the road when our lives are full of regrets. "I should have known" should not be in our vocabulary.

If you search out books on the subject, you will find many on diabetes "cures." You will also find many books published on insulin resistance "cures."

We have discussed how many of our medical problems can be at least reduced by simple dietary, nutritional, and exercise regimens. When one looks at all of the various stages of cognitive memory loss, dementia, and Alzheimer's disease, he or she needs to ask, "What steps can be taken to reverse or at least slow down this developing condition?"

It's easy to draw conclusions that cause A leads to cause B, C, and so forth. We realize it's not that simple. The best experts in the medical field are working hard to find ways to defeat these devastating diseases.

If you, a family member, or a friend has cognitive memory loss, dementia, or Alzheimer's diseases, don't battle this on your own. Seek out good medical advice and treatment. Battling long-term diseases is a marathon, not a sprint. Often those caring for family members or friends with these conditions find their own health declining over time because of fatigue, stress, and disrupted sleep patterns. We see this a lot. Our hearts go out to the patient, their family, and their friends. We find that we are looking over our shoulders hoping that someday we're not next.

The one thing we must all be aware of is that we can't live a poor lifestyle and hope that over time we can fix it with drugs. It's wonderful that there are medical remedies for diabetes, but we have to take charge of our health and do the best we can to stay healthy. That's easier said than done these days.

What you want to do is hedge your bets. In other words, don't put all your eggs in one basket. Attack the problem from as many sides as possible.

Instead of relying on one or two types of treatments to treat your inflammation, insulin resistance, prediabetes, type 2 or 3 diabetes, or even type 1 diabetes, use all of the tools at your disposal to fight the condition or disease. Use your doctor, medical caregiver, diabetes nurse or counselor, nutritionist, physical trainer, support groups, family, and friends. Don't go it alone! Ask for advice and help.

We have a tendency today to fight our battles on our own. This is the typical way to deal with our personal health problems. We must learn to fight the battle as a team.

Many conditions can be addressed by simple changes in one's life. Changes can be small and few, but over time there are significant positive results.

Never give up. We have seen what looked like hopeless situations get turned around. Ask questions of the experts. If you don't understand something, ask for explanations until you do understand it.

Help others. Helping others will help you.

# Processed Wheat, Gluten, Soy, and Sugars Can Be Toxic to Us

Endocrine-disrupting toxins—this is a term you should become familiar with. The things we eat and the things we handle can make us sick.

The foods we eat today are not the same foods that we ate even thirty years ago.

It should be no surprise that the number of diabetes cases has exploded over the past thirty years not only in the United States but worldwide.

Many foods have been genetically modified. Wheat is not the same grain as it used to be. Almost all of the soy found in the United States has been processed. The wheat and soy we eat now have a disastrous effect on our hormones, ghrelin and leptin, that control appetite.

Processed sugars, such as high-fructose corn syrup, are one of the worst things we could put into our bodies. Those, along with processed wheat gluten and soy, increase our glucose levels and create or increase our insulin resistance, which can lead to prediabetes, type 2 diabetes, and type 3 diabetes. These genetically modified foods can also lead to celiac disease, where an individual may develop IBS (irritable bowel syndrome) or even worse conditions such as Crohn's disease. If you have celiac disease, your risk of developing colon cancer is not increased by 60 percent—it's increased sixty times!

The more you can get back to food basics, the more of a chance you will have to live a longer, healthier life!

## Endocrine-Disrupting Toxins (Chemicals)

There have been foreign studies in children (China and Korea). The United States and Europe do not allow studies to be conducted with children. More and more evidence is suggesting that chemical toxins in everyday items we use, such as plastics, are interfering with the function of our internal organs and systems.

# The Five Worst Foods to Eat

- Concentrated fruit juices
- Margarine
- Whole wheat bread
- Processed soy
- Hidden processed sugars

This applies to everyone, not just diabetics!

# Senior Citizens and Type 3 Diabetes

As individuals age, their risk of developing insulin resistance (metabolic syndrome), prediabetes, or type 2 diabetes increases every year. The majority of Americans over eighty years of age have either prediabetes or type 2 diabetes. The current thinking in the medical field is that elderly people with somewhat elevated blood sugar (glucose) levels don't need any type of serious intervention to deal with this problem. Add that to the long-term use of statins (which may lead to Alzheimer's disease), and suddenly seniors may find themselves falling into the abyss of cognitive memory loss (basic reasoning ability), dementia, and Alzheimer's disease. Suddenly one may be facing one of the many faces of diabetes: type 3 diabetes!

Senior citizens find themselves attacked from all sides. Most of them have to worry about having enough money to live on. Will they someday not have enough money to pay their bills? Will they have enough medical coverage for a serious medical condition that could develop later if it hasn't already? Are they taking care of a spouse, relative, or friend, which in itself pulls down their health condition? Do they have adequate medical, social, and family guidance and supervision?

The sad fact is we live in a throwaway society. This can unfortunately apply to senior citizens. Many times intervention to help those seniors falling between the cracks must come from family members who have the authority to make critical health, financial, and housing decisions and are willing to exercise that authority. Not all seniors are fortunate enough to have someone to intervene on their behalf in a medical crisis. Social agencies, law enforcement, the private business sector, and even the medical establishment of doctors, nurses, and medical counselors along with clinics and hospitals find their hands are tied when dealing with a serious, sometimes life-threatening condition.

We all need to be proactive in watching our family and friends for the beginning signs of type 3 diabetes.

We have spent some time explaining the long journey to get to this part of one's life.

It is our hope that you choose to volunteer some of your time to helping others. We realize that many people are not senior citizens and that their lives are full of challenges and just trying to pay their bills and keep their heads above water.

For those of us fortunate enough to be able to carve out some time in our schedules, we need to make a conscious decision what impact we want to make to help our fellow humans. What's the best cause to join?

The one you have a passion for!

We would certainly encourage you to step out of your comfort zone.

When we give presentations to groups about the various types of diabetes, including type 3 diabetes, the reaction of the audience is almost a stunned disbelief. The information is powerful and frightening. The older the person in the audience is, the more the concern shows on their face.

We discuss the various forms of diabetes to all ages of patients. Certainly the sooner one can take precautions to prevent getting prediabetes or type 2 or type 3 diabetes, the better. Senior patients don't have a lot of time to fix the problem of diabetes. Unfortunately not all medical professionals take elevated blood sugar (glucose) levels seriously in elderly patients. You as a patient (or a family member on your behalf) must ask questions of your doctor, diabetes counselor, and other medical advisers and insist you get answers that satisfy your concerns. Keep pressing until you feel like you are in charge of your health destiny. Remember that your health and your *life* may be on the line.

Once again, remember that helping others will help you. We have sat in sessions as attendees and sometimes have come away with valuable information we can use and share with others.

Start thinking in terms of type 3 diabetes.

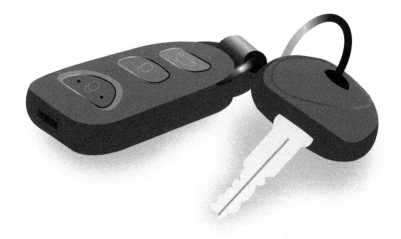

# The Keys to the Car

If you understand pH balance, inflammation, and insulin resistance and take steps to prevent or reverse these conditions, you can potentially overcome *any* of the major life-threatening health conditions that exist today.

You will have the keys to the car and will be in the driver's seat with regard to your health.

Your body is like a finely tuned sports car. Don't give it cheap gas, oil, and fluids. Give it the best!

# Questions and Answers

Q: Can I eat after eight in the evening?

A: Yes, if you haven't exceeded your calorie intake for the day. You don't want to eat processed carbohydrates and sugars after eight o'clock.

Q: Will resistance training help me lower my glucose levels?

A: *Yes.* Prediabetes and type 2 diabetes patients who use resistance training are seeing reduced glucose levels. Combine that with low-resistance interval training, and you have a powerful weapon against diabetes. It is recommended that you have a fifteen-gram serving of protein within forty-five minutes of finishing your morning exercise routine. This will help your muscle cells to repair themselves and should help you in weight loss if you're attempting that.

Q: How many calories should I eat each day?

A: Ask your doctor. Set targets and goals with your doctor. You can go online and review the calorie guides put out by the US government. We often tend to underestimate the number of calories we take in and overestimate the amount of exercise we do. Don't set your calorie intake too low! Your body will save the calories for protection.

Q: Should I avoid fast food?

A: Yes, avoid fast food at all times. It will turn to sugar fast. Also, the saturated fat level is very high, along with high sodium levels, which is bad for your blood pressure.

Q: What are the benefits if any of capsaicin?

A: There are definite health benefits for diabetes patients. It slows the release of insulin by about thirty minutes. This compound is found in chili peppers.

Generally you will see cayenne pepper and not chili pepper put into capsules you take. Hot spicy foods tend to rev up our metabolism. Capsaicin is found in peppers such as jalapeno peppers. Ingesting capsaicin will slow the release of insulin by about thirty minutes. Twelve thousand micrograms or 120,000 thermal units (in pill form) is the average recommended dosage for most people. Check with your doctor *before* starting to consume capsaicin.

Q: Does metabolism or the burning of calories really change much whether I'm sitting down or casually moving?

A: Once you sit down, your metabolism immediately slows down to just a single calorie burn per minute.

# Summary

It is our sincerest hope that you review our first book, *The Diabetes Slayer's Handbook: Preventing or Reversing Prediabetes and Type 2 Diabetes*. In this book, we have built on the concepts of that book and gone out much further in our delivery of ideas and effective approaches to fight the deadly disease called diabetes.

You have probably noticed our food charts are full of items that are anti-inflammatory, low in poor-quality preservatives and processed carbohydrates and sugars, and are gluten-free. By slowing and blocking the carbohydrates being absorbed in your bloodstream and burning and neutralizing sugars and increasing your metabolic rate, you create an effective opposition to insulin resistance, prediabetes, and type 2 and type 3 diabetes. Lower carbohydrate intake, to start with, will help a lot. An increased intake of chlorophyll (eating green) helps to greatly reduce insulin resistance by reducing cell inflammation and swelling. Add low-resistance interval training along with weight training and resistance training, and you should start seeing results and feeling better immediately.

Type 3 diabetes is a term you won't hear much right now, but over the coming years, you will hear about it. If you take the right steps, you may be able to prevent or at least delay contracting this new form of diabetes—dementia and Alzheimer's disease.

As a final observation, studies are indicating that people who die from heart attacks and strokes have one reoccurring factor or marker that shows, and that is elevated blood sugars!

# Conclusion

Both of us authors have battled diabetes over the years, from type 1 diabetes to prediabetes and type 2 diabetes. In addition, we have worked alongside diabetic patients and their families and their friends. This has helped us deal better with our approach to good health regardless of external circumstances and conditions.

We'd like to clear the air about diabetes patients being responsible for their state of health. No, they are *not* lazy, fat, and reckless with their health. Many of these people developed this disease because of genetics and circumstances. Give these people the medical knowledge they deserve to have, along with support from family, friends, and support groups, plus their medical caregivers and counselors, and they will generally do well for themselves. Many diabetes patients are busy caring for spouses, family members, or friends who are seriously ill. That alone takes a toll on their own personal health.

We have gone through the long chain of conditions of high body acid levels, inflammation, insulin resistance, prediabetes, various stages of type 2 diabetes, and the final threat of eventually type 3 diabetes. Every effort is being made to find a cure for these various forms of diabetes, and much research and development has occurred. And more will occur.

Helping others will help you have a reason to get up in the morning.

Have somewhere to go every day—the gym, your place of worship, library, senior center, diabetes education classes, your job, volunteer work, even going for a walk or working in your yard.

Get a desk or wall calendar, and plan out each month in advance. Think into the future. Where do you want to be in five, ten, or fifteen years from now? Forget about how you used to look back in high school or college. Sometimes going to a high school reunion can be beneficial for you. If you think you look bad, get a load of how the other guys look now! If you don't have an immediate family member or spouse, team up with a friend and join an organization; a club, hobby, or craft that involves other people who have similar interests to yours. Getting in contact with other people helps to start to set the wellness stage.

It is the option of us authors that preventative measures, exercise, and diabetes reversal techniques can help to prevent, slow, or in some cases reverse some states of diabetes. Diabetes reversal is *not a cure*, but it's a great alternative.

We must *never give up* fighting diabetes.

How we conduct our lives influences those around us. Helping others in turn helps us. Diabetes patients, their families, and friends give us strength and determination to continue our efforts to get the message out that the concepts of integrated medicine and complementary alternative medicine have a place in our society. Faith plays a very important role in our wellness. Sometimes we need to be reminded that healing starts from deep within ourselves. Regardless of your belief or disbelief of a higher power influencing our lives, there is an inner soul or core within us that connects to the quantum universe. This is everything that was ever, is, or will be. If you believe, you can achieve.

In our previous book, *The Diabetes Slayer's Handbook: Preventing or Reversing Prediabetes and Type 2 Diabetes*, we wanted the reader to come away with one piece of advice. Diabetes is a terrorist. It will maim and kill as many innocent people as it can—over sixty thousand Americans per year. *You do not negotiate with a terrorist!*

Remember that from adversity comes opportunity. Both of us authors have experienced health setbacks. From those setbacks we have rebounded stronger than ever. We don't pretend to have all of the answers for maintaining good health or improving poor health to a better level.

Much of what happens to us is from our own actions. It's not so much what happens to us but what we do to respond to it.

We think of the story of someone who received a free gift and complained that the gift needed some repairs done to it. They were told of the person who asked for help to "dig themselves out." The next morning they woke up to see a garden shovel next to their bed. In other words, we have to put out some effort to help ourselves. "Some assembly required" comes to mind.

What will our legacy be after we are gone? Did we help others? Did others help us? We are all in this health battle together. There is a responsibility for us to make a difference. We believe in the goodness of humanity. Never should we lose sight of the gift of life we received. Make every day count!

Live well, our friends.

The Turtle

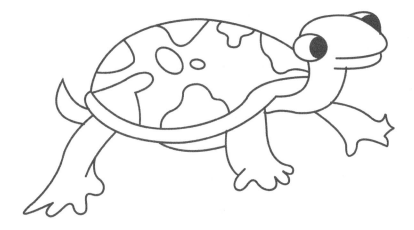

Slow and Steady wins the game

# Our Mission

The mission of the Diabetes Information Group (DIG) is to empower patients with the means, the will, and the knowledge to combat and defeat diabetes.

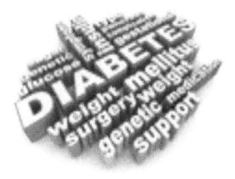

The organization was cofounded in May 2014 by Maria Lizotte, RN, BSN, and CDE, along with Alan D. Raguso, volunteer peer group educator and published author.

The group is financially self-sufficient and does not ask for donations. Medical referrals are not required in order to attend the meetings. Attendance is free of charge, as are handouts and provided information. The meetings are open to prediabetics and type 1 and type 2 diabetics, along with their families and friends.

Maria Lizotte has many years of experience in diabetes education, including from the University of Pittsburgh Medical Center, Disetronic Diabetes Corp., Joslin Diabetes Center / Clara Barton Camps, Cedars Sinai Medical Center, Medtronic Insulin Pump Certified Trainer, Animas Corp Certified Insulin Pump Trainer, UCLA, and Walla Walla General Hospital. Maria has nutrition expertise in weight loss, diabetes / high blood sugars, celiac, Crohn's, and IBS diet food sensitivities, allergies, autoimmune disease diet, low-carbohydrate high-fat diet, and hypoglycemia diet.

Alan D. Raguso is a published author who speaks to fellow patients with knowledge that helps fight diabetes. His book is *given free to those who cannot afford to buy it.*

Both Lizotte and Raguso lecture free of charge *because it's the right thing to do.* They provide critical medical knowledge that's given free of charge to the public.

The Diabetes Information Group (The DIG) Mission
Statement, Copyright, May 2014

# About the Author

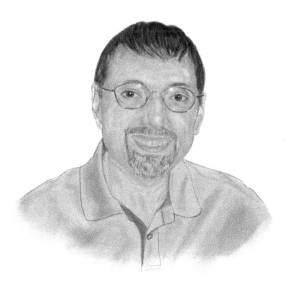

## Alan D. Raguso

In January 2001 Raguso was diagnosed with type 2 diabetes. He struggled with the condition for years. Finally in 2010 he took steps to improve his health based on practical and effective methods for weight loss and glucose reduction. On October 12, 2012, he published *The Diabetes Slayer's Handbook: Preventing or Reversing Prediabetes and Type 2 Diabetes*.

Alan has been a member of the advisory committee for diabetes education at Providence St. Mary Medical Center for more than five years. He also participated in the local YMCA On the Edge program. On May 5, 2014, Alan Raguso and Maria Lizotte formed the DIG (the Diabetes Information Group). Alan and Maria hold monthly diabetes support group meetings for prediabetics and types 1 and 2 diabetics. Alan also participates in presentations at SonBridge Community Services Center.

Alan is a graduate of Washington State University.

Raguso is retired and resides in Washington State. Some of his other interests are collecting old rock-and-roll records, astronomy, and enjoying vintage collectible cars.

# About the Author

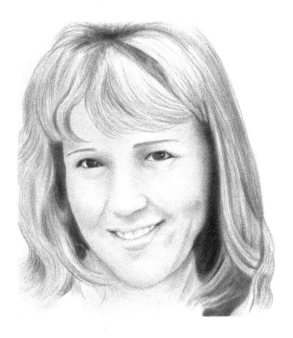

## Maria Lizotte

Maria Lizotte has a bachelor's degree in nursing from the University of Pittsburgh. She originally trained through the Joslin Diabetes Center in Boston and has been teaching as a certified diabetes educator since 1993. Originally from California, Maria worked for the diabetes and endocrinology centers at both Cedars-Sinai Medical Center and UCLA before coming to Walla Walla. Maria has been lecturing on diabetes for local TV and radio. She is a guest speaker for and a member of Providence St. Mary Medical Center Advisory Committee for Diabetes Education. Having lived with diabetes since 1985, she has a unique understanding of what people with diabetes live with and a desire to share her knowledge to aid others dealing with the disease.

Whether you have prediabetes, are at risk for diabetes, or are already diagnosed, these lectures will help all who are interested in learning how to reverse insulin resistance and enjoy an excellent quality of life despite diabetes. Volunteering with Maria is Alan Raguso. A lifelong Walla Walla resident, Alan recently published his own story, titled *The Diabetes Slayer's Handbook: Preventing or Reversing Prediabetes and Type 2 Diabetes*, about reversing his type 2 diabetes to support others on the same journey. Both Alan and Maria donate their time and experience to helping others avoid kidney failure, blindness, and heart and nerve damage from the disease.

# Resources

Agatston, Arthur. *The South Beach Diet Good Fats Good Carbs Guide*. Emmaus, PA: Rodale Press, 2004.

Alzheimer's Assoc. National Capital Area Chapter
8180 Greensboro Drive
Suite 400
McLean, VA 22102

American Association of Diabetes Educators, AADE
(Local Diabetes Educator Referral System)
444 North Michigan Ave.
Suite 1240
Chicago, Il 60611
www.diabeteseducator.org/diabeteseducation/definitions.html

American Diabetes Association
1660 Duke St.
Alexandria, VA 22314
www.diabeteseducator.org

Bernstein, Richard K. *The Diabetes Miracle*. Boston: Little, Brown & Co., 2011.

CHOICES Health Education & Wellness Program. "Get the Most Out of Your Workout in the Shortest Possible Time! *Interval Training* 1, no. 2 (August–September 2008).

"Does Vinegar Control Type 2 Diabetes?—A List of Acidic Foods to Help Lower Blood Sugar Levels." Beverleigh H. Piepers. www.Ezlnearticles.com.

"Effects of Exercise Training Intensity on Pancreatic B-Cell Function." *Diabetes Care* 32, no. 10 (October 2009).

"Foods That Reduce Blood Glucose/Livestrong.com." www.livestrong.com/article/3535 07-foods-that-reduce-blood-glucose/.

Germa, Maria M. Adeva (Souto). "Diet Induced Metabolic Acidosis." *Clinical Nutrition* 30, no. 4 (August 2011): 416–421.
*First for Women* (August 12, 2013): 60–63.
Sss.diabetes.co.uk/news2014/may weds 14, May 2014.

Glycemic Load Index
David Mendosa
93 E. Moorhead Cir. Suite 2F
Boulder, Colorado 80305
mendosa@mendosa.com

Good Nutrition: Should Guidelines Differ for Men and Women)?"
The Harvard Medical School
www.health.harvard.edu

Gotthardt, Melissa. "Melt Off Fat." *First for Women* (July 18, 2011): 28–35.

———. "Body Weight Set-Point Discovery. *First for Women* (October 10, 2011): 32–37.

———. "The Day-Off Secret That Melts Stubborn Body Fat." *First for Women* (October 31, 2011): 32–37.

———. "Soup Melts Away 10X More Weight." *First for Women* (January 23, 2012): 32–35.

———. "Discover Your Mind/Body Secret." *First for Women* (February 13, 2012): 32–37.

———. "European Secret Triples Weight Loss." *First for Women* (April 29, 2013): 30–35.

———. "Walking Cures for Hormonal Belly Fat." *First for Women* (May 20, 2013): 40–43.

———. "Outsmart Insulin Bumps & Fat Just Falls Off!" *First for Women* (September 2, 2013): 26–29.

———. "Wheat-Free Living Melts Stubborn Fat." *First for Women* (January 6, 2014): 60–69.

Greenfield, Paige. "Make Over Your Metabolism." *Health* (January/February 2012): 45–50.

Hiser, Elizabeth. *The Other Diabetes*. New York: William Morrow & Co., Inc., 1999.

Institute for Dementia Research & Prevention / Pennington Biomedical Research Center
6400 Perkins Road
Baton Rouge, LA 70808

Joslin Blog, September 23, 2011, by Joslin Communications.

Krames Patient Education. "Living Well with Diabetes." 2011. baypines. kramesonline.com/LivingWellWithType2Diabetes.

Lowenstein, Kate. "The Burning Question." *Health* (November 2011): 24 and 95.

Maxbauer, L. "How Doctors Lose Weight." *First for Women* (August 29, 2011): 36–41.

Mayo Clinic. *Solutions for Living with Diabetes*. New York: Oxmoor House, 2015.

Nutrition Graphics
P. O. Box 276264
Sacramento, CA 95827
www.ngcatalog.com

Purlmutter, David. *Grain Brain*. Boston: Little, Brown & Co., 2013.

Raguso, Alan D. *The Diabetes Slayer's Handbook: Preventing or Reversing Prediabetes and Type 2 Diabetes*. Bloomington, IN: iUniverse Press, 2012.

Shaw, Gina. "You Can Beat the Big D." *Health* (November 2011): 95.

Sidorov, Max. 7 Steps to Health. Victoria, BC, Canada: The ICTM Organization, 2014.

Solan, Michael, and Melissa Gotthardt. "Nutrient Combos That Melt Super Stubborn Fat." *First for Women* (December 12, 2011): 28–33.

World Health Organization
Avenue Appia 20
1211
Geneva 27

# Index

## A

A1C
described, 22
    in people with prediabetes, 14
    in people with type 2 diabetes, 18
    possible causes and possible
        responses to higher than
        normal A1C, 49
    recommended level of, 62
A1C/eAG conversion chart, 63
ABS, 40
acid-forming foods, recommended
    dietary intake of, 12
acidic diet, pickle as acidic, 32
acidity, cautions with, 12
activity, recommendation for, 55
adult onset diabetes. *See* type 2
    diabetes
advice/help, importance of asking
    for, 82
alcohol, 25
alkaline diet
    benefits of, 22, 23, 31
    cucumber as alkaline, 32
    described, 43–44, 80
alkaline substances, 36
alkaline-forming foods,
    recommended dietary intake
    of, 12
Alzheimer's disease

possible connections to of statins,
    40, 85
type 3 diabetes possibly resulting
    in, 2, 19, 80, 81, 85
amputation of toes, feet, and legs, 14
antibodies, as testing marker, 1, 77
antioxidants, 53
appetite attacks, possible causes and
    possible responses to, 49
apple peel, 67
aspartame, 68, 76
autoimmune disease
    LADA (latent autoimmune
        diabetes of adults) as, 16
    type 1 diabetes as, 15
Avastin, use of on vision problems, 34

## B

B complex vitamins/B vitamins. *See*
    *also specific B vitamins*, 51, 67
balance, importance of, 30–31
balance training, 71
beef, minerals and vitamins in, 60
BEST syndrome, 39–42
beta cell failure, in people with type
    1.5 diabetes, 16
biological factors in diabetes, 40
biomarkers, 77–78
biotin, 67
blood pressure
    high blood pressure as part of
        metabolic syndrome, 13

possible causes and possible responses to high blood pressure, 50

blood sugar
excess levels of as causing long-term cognitive memory loss, 19
goals for, 57
high blood sugar as end cause of all damage to body and brain, 16
monitoring of, 34

blood vessel scarring in the eye, 34

BMI (body mass index), 52

body density composition, 52

BPA, 40

## C

C peptide, as testing marker, 1, 77

caffeine, cautions with, 21

calcium, foods with, 59

calcium supplement, 21

calories
how many to eat, 88
saving, 67

capsaicin, benefits of, 46, 50, 72, 88–89

carbohydrates
dense carbohydrates, 34, 45, 74
fast carbohydrates, 28
as food group, 24
and glycemic load, 61
high-carbohydrate diet, 19
limiting intake of bad carbohydrates, 12
low-carbohydrate diet, 16, 44, 58–60
moderate carbohydrates, 28
natural carbohydrates, 45, 74
processed carbohydrates, 19, 20, 26, 31, 33, 45, 48, 54, 55, 74, 76, 88

recommended dietary intake of, 26
slow carbohydrates, 28
three states of, 27, 28–29

celiac disease, 83

cheese, minerals and vitamins in, 60

chlorophyll, benefits of, 20, 25, 33, 45–46, 55

chocolate, 54, 56

chromium, 34, 56, 59

cinnamon, 54, 56

circulation problems, 14

CMP (Comprehensive Metabolic Profile), 56

coconut oil, 33, 34

cod liver oil, 33

cognitive memory loss (CML), 19, 78, 81, 82, 85

companionship, importance of, 8, 9

convergence, 79

copper, 51, 60

cortisol, 72

Crohn's disease, 83

## D

dawn phenomenon, 20

death, diabetic conditions as leading to, 31

debilitation, diabetic conditions as leading to, 31

dementia
possible connections to of statins, 40
type 3 diabetes possibly resulting in, 2, 19, 80, 81, 85

diabetes. *See also specific types*
annual deaths caused by, 7
coping with as not acceptable, 9
forms of, 1
increase in cases of, 83
as reversible but never gone, 6

as rooted in genetics, lifestyle, and environmental influences, 6

as terrorist, 7, 94

Diabetes Information Group (DIG), 97

diabetes mellitus. *See* type 2 diabetes

*The Diabetes Slayer's Handbook* (Raguso), 2, 6, 7, 54, 94

diet, role of for people with type 2 diabetes, 18

diet drinks, cautions with, 55

dietary fiber, 66

diseases. *See also specific diseases*

battling long-term diseases as marathon, not sprint, 82

body chemistry link to, 3–5

**E**

economic factors in diabetes, 40–41

egg, minerals and vitamins in, 60

endocrine disruptors/endocrine-disrupting toxins, 17, 83

environmental factors in diabetes, 40

environmental toxins, 16

excess weight

as part of metabolic syndrome, 13

possible causes and possible responses to, 49

as possible contributing factor to type 2 diabetes, 18

exercise

balance training, 71

benefits of, 33

consulting with medical professionals before starting any exercise program, 70

importance of timing regarding, 74

Low-Resistance Interval Training (LRIT), 49, 50

resistance training, 33, 55, 70–71

role of for people with type 2 diabetes, 18

weight training, 70, 71

eye disease, 14

**F**

family, diabetic conditions as leading to strains on, 31

fast carbohydrates, 28

fast food, 88

fasting glucose levels

in people with prediabetes, 14

in people with type 2 diabetes, 18

fat loss, certain proteins as accelerating, 11

fats, 25, 33, 34

ferritin, testing for, 56

fiber

benefits of, 33, 34

dietary fiber, 66

in green leafy vegetables, 25

fiber and acidics (FAA), 64

fish oil, 33, 34

flavonols, 54, 56

flax oil, 33, 34

fluorine, 59

folate (vitamin B9), 52, 59

folic acid, 52, 56

food arsenal, stocking, 66–68

food groups

alcohol, 25

carbohydrates, 24

fats, 25

fruits, 24–25

milk, 25

nonstarchy vegetables, 25

proteins, 25

sweets, desserts, and other carbohydrates, 25

food labels, importance of reading, 20, 26, 33, 65

foods
 five worst foods to eat, 84
 that are diabetic friendly, 75

foot neuropathy, 34

four Bs, 50, 64

friends, diabetic conditions as leading to strains on, 31

fruits, 24–25

# G

genetic markers, 77

genetically modified foods, 83

genetics, 77–78

gestational diabetes, 1, 2

GH (growth hormone), 73

ghrelin, 72, 83

glucagon, 72

glucose bumps, 21, 22, 27

glucose levels
 importance of checking, 14
 importance of regulating postmeal glucose levels, 20
 maintaining low glucose levels, 62–63
 in people with prediabetes, 14
 possible causes and possible responses to higher than normal glucose levels, 49

glucose spikes, 20, 21, 22

glucose stability, 22

glucose variability, 22

glycemic load, 35, 48, 61, 69, 75–76

glycemic tables, 33

glycosuria, 51

grapefruit, as working to neutralize toxic acids in body, 27, 80

grazing, 33, 74

green leafy vegetables, benefits of, 25

growth hormone (GH), 73

# H

HDL
 low HDL as part of metabolic syndrome, 13
 possible causes and possible responses to low HDL, 50

heart attacks, 14

hGH or HGH (human growth hormone), 73

high acidic levels, consequences of, 81

high-acid substances, 36–38

high-alkaline diet, as helping reverse insulin resistance, 23

high-carbohydrate diet, as one of cause of type 2 and type 3 diabetes, 19

high-fructose corn syrups, cautions with, 21, 83

high-pH diet, 80

homocysteine and fasting insulin lab, 56

homocystinuria, 78

hormones. *See also specific hormones,* 2, 22, 56, 72–73, 83

human growth hormone (hGH or HGH), 73

hydrogen, definition of power of, 35

hyperglycemia, 51, 53

hypoglycemia, 28

# I

IBS (irritable bowel syndrome), 83

inflammation, consequences of, 12, 13, 81

insulin
 production of, 72
 release of, 72
 role of, 22

insulin injection, for people with type 1 diabetes, 15

insulin resistance, 1, 12, 13, 22–23, 70, 81
interval training, 33, 49, 50
iron, 51, 59

**J**

joint pain, possible causes and possible responses to, 50

**K**

kidney disease, 14, 51
kidney scarring, 34

**L**

labs to ask for, 56
LADA (latent autoimmune diabetes of adults), 1, 16
laser surgery, use of on vision problems, 34
LDL
    "bad" cholesterol, 4
    "dense" LDL, 4
    "fluffy" LDL, 4
    high LDL as part of metabolic syndrome, 13
    possible causes and possible responses to higher than normal LDL, 50
lemons, as working to neutralize toxic acids in body, 12, 27, 80
leptin, 72, 83
limes, as working to neutralize toxic acids in body, 27, 80
Lizotte, Maria, personal story of type 1 diabetes, 10
low-carbohydrate diet, 16, 44, 58–60
low-density "fast" carbohydrates, 28
low–glycemic load foods, 69, 75–76
Low-Resistance Interval Training (LRIT), 49, 50

**M**

magnesium, 21, 53–54, 56, 59
manganese, 51, 60
marker, defined, 77
medical costs, diabetic conditions as leading to exorbitant medical costs, 31
Medicare Advantage insurance plan, 23
Mediterranean anti-inflammation diet (MAID), 12, 25, 26, 43, 45–46, 49, 55
metabolic syndrome, 13, 22, 85
metabolism
    benefits of increasing, 20
    defined, 50
    effects on of sitting down or casually moving, 89
    grazing as increasing, 74
    spices as increasing, 69, 75–76
    vitamins B1, B12, and biotin as increasing, 67
metformin, 1, 55, 56
methionine, 78
methyl cycle, 78
methylfolate (vitamin B9), 78
micronutrients, 51
milk, 25
minerals. *See also specific minerals*, 33, 51
moderate carbohydrates, 28
moderate–glycemic load foods, 75–76
MODY (maturity onset of diabetes in youth), 1, 16
MTHFR gene, 52, 78
MTHFR lab, 56

**N**

natural foods, pH factor in, 12
natural sugar, compared to refined/ processed sugar, 12

nerve disease, 14
neutral substances, 35
nonfasting glucose levels, in people
    with prediabetes, 14
nonstarchy vegetables, 25

## O

oils, recommended ones, 33
olive oil, 33, 34
omega-3 fats, 25, 31, 45, 50, 59, 72, 74
omega-6 fats, 25, 31, 50
overacidity, as triggering weight
    gain, 12

## P

pantothenic acid, 60
peripheral neuropathy, 34
personal training plan, 70
pH, defined, 35
pH balance, 11–12, 31, 35
pH levels, 80–82
phosphorous, 59
phytochemicals, 67
plastics, 17, 33, 40, 83
plate balance, 74
potassium, 59
prediabetes
    described, 14
    as form of diabetes, 1
    insulin resistance as precursor to,
        13, 81
    no diagnosis of in 2000, 81
    statistics on Americans over
        sixty-five having, 52
prescription drugs, as potentially
    causing insulin resistance, 23
processed carbohydrates, 19, 20, 26,
    31, 33, 45, 48, 54, 55, 74, 76, 88
proteins, 1, 11, 25, 26, 31, 34, 44, 45,
    46, 48, 49, 58, 72, 74, 78, 79, 88

## Q

quality of life, diabetic conditions as
    leading to reduction in, 31
questions and answers, 88–89

## R

RBC (Red Blood Cell) lab, 56
    refined/processed sugar
        cautions with, 12, 33, 83
        counting of, 48
repetitions (reps), 70
resistance training, 33, 55, 70–71, 88
retinopathy, 34
reversal techniques (for diabetes),
    33–34

## S

"Safe" House food guide, 44, 45, 47, 55
selenium, 51, 60
senior citizens, and type 3 diabetes,
    85–86
serum vitamin C, 51
serving size, 29
sex hormones, testing for, 56
slow carbohydrates, 28
social factors in diabetes, 41
sodium, 59
Somatotropine, 73
soy, processed, 83
spicy/hot foods, benefits of. See also
    capsaicin, 46
starches, 28, 29
statins
    as one possible source of elevated
        glucose resistance, 23
    possible connections to dementia
        and Alzheimer's, 40, 85
steamroller illustration, 7, 9
steroids, use of on vision problems, 34
stevia, 12, 33, 34

stroke, 14
Styrofoam, 40
sucralose, 67, 68, 75, 76
sugar alcohols, 24, 48, 69
sugar substitutes, 12, 68
sugar-free products, 67, 69, 75
sugars
    acidics as neutralizing, 64
    defined, 35
    importance of timing and control
        consumption of, 20
    refined/processed sugar, 12, 33,
        48, 83
supplements. *See also specific
    supplements*
    benefits of mineral supplement,
        33, 34
    calcium supplement, 21
    doses of for insulin resistance, 56
sweets, desserts, and other
    carbohydrates, 25

T

technological factors in diabetes,
    41–42
test strips, 22–23
three Ps, 50, 65
"The Three Mirrors," 3, 5, 13
timing, importance of, 74
tissue pain, possible causes and
    possible responses to, 50
total diabetes warfare, 6–8, 31
toxins, 16, 17, 22, 40, 46, 77, 83
trace elements, 51
triglyceride levels
    high triglyceride levels as part of
        metabolic syndrome, 13
    possible causes and possible
        responses to higher than
        normal triglycerides, 50
type 1 diabetes

described, 15
as form of diabetes, 1
genetics and biomarkers for, 77
no cure for at this time, 80
type 1.5 diabetes
    described, 16–17
    as form of diabetes, 1
type 2 diabetes
    add odds of developing dementia
        or Alzheimer's disease, 81
    described, 2, 18
    as form of diabetes, 1
    genetics and biomarkers for, 77
    no cure for at this time, 80
type 3 diabetes. *See also* Alzheimer's
    disease; *also* dementia
    described, 2, 19
    as form of diabetes, 1
    senior citizens and, 85–86
    use of term, 55

V

vitamin A, 51, 58, 60
vitamin B1, 58, 67
vitamin B2, 58
vitamin B3, 58
vitamin B5, 58
vitamin B6, 58, 60
vitamin B7, 58
vitamin B9 (folate), 52, 59, 78
vitamin B12, 34, 52, 55, 56, 59, 60, 67
vitamin C, 34, 49, 51, 52–53, 56, 59, 72
vitamin D, 49, 51–52, 55, 59, 60
vitamin D3, 34, 52, 67
vitamin E, 34, 51, 59
vitamin K, 59
vitamin receptors (VDRs), 51
vitamins, in general, 51

## W

water, 27
weight gain, overacidity as
       triggering, 12
weight training, 70, 71
wheat, processed, 83

## Z

zinc, 53, 56, 59

CPSIA information can be obtained
at www.ICGtesting.com
Printed in the USA
LVHW100236020622
720309LV00004B/56